HOME REMEDIES ℞

How to Use This Book

When you're not feeling quite up to par and want a remedy that works and is made with ingredients you already have around the house, it's time to reach for *Home Remedies Rx*. Especially if the last thing you want to fit into your day is a trip to the doctor or pharmacy. Inside these pages you'll find help for common everyday ailments, personal and body care, baby and childcare, techniques for prenatal wellness, and even remedies for your pets.

This easy-to-use book will help you sort out the difference between old wives' tales, urban legends, and real remedies that work—with explanations of the science behind the most effective treatments for common ailments.

Home Remedies Rx is divided into three sections:

Part I: Understanding Home Remedies (page 1–19)

Here you'll learn the basics of home remedies, from their origins in the earliest days of recorded history to how to use the vast availability of ingredients you'll need today.

Part II: Healing Foods, Household Products, and Essential Oils (page 21–97)

In this section, you'll discover what to keep on hand in your kitchen cupboard or medicine cabinet, so you can reach for the right herb, spice, essence, or object when you need relief. You'll be surprised at the number of items you already have around the house that have healing properties. With this knowledge in hand, you will spend less money to feel better faster.

Part III: Everyday Home Remedies (page 99–288)

What should you use for a headache, earache, tummy ache, or eyestrain? How should you treat a common cold, the flu, or your child's case of croup? What are the best beauty remedies for acne, puffy eyes, and wrinkles? This book gives you more than 500 simple remedies to treat what ails you and your family, making this your go-to guide whenever someone in your household needs a little help to feel better.

Home Remedies Rx may revolutionize the way you approach wellness and healing in your family, providing the instructions you need to eliminate many expensive over-the-counter medicines and replace them with natural tools that work.

HOME REMEDIES

Rx

DIY Prescriptions When You Need Them Most

ALTHEA
PRESS

Contents

vii Foreword

viii Introduction

PART I

I **Understanding Home Remedies**

3 1 The Basics of Home Remedies

13 2 Getting Started with Home Remedies

PART II

21 **Healing Foods, Household Products, and Essential Oils**

22 3 Healing Foods

52 4 Healing Household Products

76 5 Healing Essential Oils

PART III

98 **Everyday Home Remedies**

100 6 Common Everyday Ailments

198 7 Prenatal, Baby, and Child-Age Ailments

240 8 Everyday Wellness & Grooming

278 9 Common Pet Ailments

289 Glossary

292 How to Build a Home Remedy First Aid Kit

293 References

301 Ailments Index

303 Index

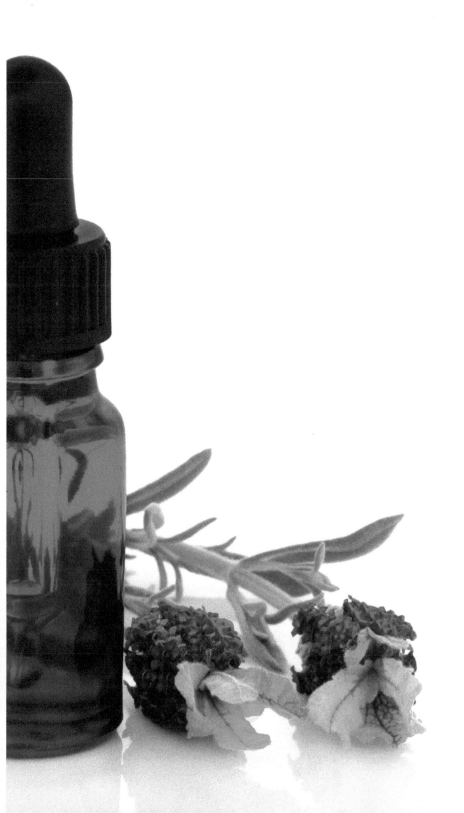

Foreword

Natural remedies are truly amazing. Not only will they save you time and money, but you will also be impressed by how well they actually work! It's incredible how a few things from your pantry can alleviate an upset stomach, a runny nose, bug bites, migraines, and even tangled hair.

I am truly impressed with *Home Remedies Rx*. It is a wealth of information, covering everything from using essential oils responsibly to dealing with daily aches and pains; there is even a section with natural remedies for your pets! A few personal favorites of mine include using peppermint, which can ease a headache, and ginger root, which can be made into tea to calm an upset stomach.

Natural remedies are great alternatives to conventional treatment since you know exactly what you are putting on or into your body. This wisdom from generations before us has been passed down for a reason: because it works.

This book is a responsible guide for beginners, a great resource for natural remedy veterans, and a perfect addition to your healthy living bookshelf!

Healthy wishes to you and yours,

Katie Peters
GIRLMEETSNOURISHMENT.COM

Introduction

It's 3 a.m., and your little one wakes up with all the symptoms of an ear infection. She can't go back to sleep. There's nowhere to go in the middle of the night to get a prescription filled—even if you could reach your pediatrician. With your child whimpering in your arms, you head to the kitchen. What can you do to make her feel better?

Inside the pantry you find your answer. You pour a little olive oil in a glass bowl and heat it up for twenty seconds in the microwave oven. Using an eyedropper, you place just a few drops of the warm liquid in your daughter's ear. The soothing oil works its way into her ear canal, and in a few minutes, your child is looking around for something to do. The pain is gone! She sits up and you let the oil drain out onto a cotton ball. Minutes later, she's back in bed and going to sleep . . . and so are you. No emergency room visit, no doctor bills, and no prescriptions.

Simple home remedies like this one have been passed down for generations—perhaps for millennia. Since humans began making tools and gathering roots and berries, home remedies have been a necessary and valuable part of our existence. Many may seem like homespun traditions, but a remarkable number of home remedies have a solid basis in science, and laboratory research has borne out the healing properties both in plants and plant-based substances like herbs and spices, essential oils derived from natural sources, and in the most basic health advice: get more rest, more exercise, and more nutrients from the food you eat.

Why have home remedies risen to the top of public consciousness recently? Perhaps it's the high cost of health care and prescriptions that have driven many families back to their roots, and the simple solutions that Grandma used. When the choice is between paying a $120 dermatology bill or taping a freshly cut half of a garlic clove to a wart on a finger, many people are more than willing to try out the garlic.

Not only are many of the ingredients used in home remedies also found in pharmaceuticals, but increasingly, the use of home remedies are being supported by modern science, making them viable alternatives to doctor visits. Let's look closely at that wart and garlic: A study conducted in a medical research laboratory and published in the *Journal of Dermatology* found that garlic works in reducing and removing warts. Now we know that the garlic contains antifungal and antiviral agents that work against the human papilloma virus (HPV) that causes warts. When the next wart appears, you'll reach for the garlic again with confidence, instead of paying for a liquid-nitrogen treatment or using an acid-based medicine.

Home remedies are not always a cure; in fact, most can only treat the symptoms of an illness or condition. Some remedies, such as for pinkeye, may take a few days to work, but most should bring you relief with a few hours. If they don't, or if you have symptoms of infection or a more serious illness, you should always default to your primary care physician.

Use *Home Remedies Rx* like a reference book. Take some time to review part 1, which will help you understand what home remedies are and how they work. In part 2, you'll learn about key foods that contribute to your health and well-being, and about those foods with healing properties, as well. After all, the best way to maintain wellness is to prevent yourself and your family from getting sick.

In part 2 you will also learn about household products and a range of essential oils that help with healing and wellness. The remedies in this section are arranged in an easy-to-follow A-to-Z format, allowing you to find what you're looking for quickly.

In part 3, you'll find information about hundreds of remedies for specific illnesses and conditions, also arranged alphabetically for easy reference. The "Why It Works" tips in this section will help you understand the science behind the remedy, and the advice on "When to See a Doctor" will bolster your confidence and good judgment on when to use a home remedy and when you should seek professional medical advice.

You've picked up this book because you know that you have—or should have—many options when it comes to your medical care. Wanting the best for yourself and your family doesn't always mean a trip to the doctor. The hundreds of simple, natural home remedies in this book are safe, affordable options that you can administer from the comfort of your home. Healing power isn't limited to the medical establishment; it's in your hands now.

At its heart, *Home Remedies Rx* is like an insurance policy. Ideally, you'll never need to use it. But if you do, the information you need is at your fingertips to enable you to act quickly and with confidence to ameliorate and eliminate the everyday problems that slow us down.

The Editors of Althea Press

PART I

UNDERSTANDING HOME REMEDIES

1 The Basics of Home Remedies

2 Getting Started with Home Remedies

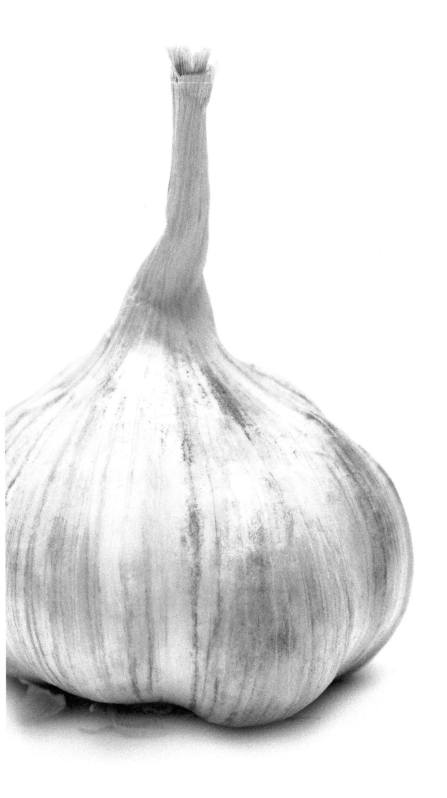

CHAPTER 1

The Basics of Home Remedies

Feeling unwell on occasion is part of the human experience, and we can't avoid the scrapes and bumps that come with physical activity, or the aches and pains of overexertion, carrying a child, playing a sport, or growing older. What we can avoid, however, is making every new symptom a reason to pay a doctor and a pharmacy for something to make us feel better.

Finding the remedies we need at home seems like a lost art, but it's one that has grown in popularity in recent years. Today people have the opportunity to share their insights and results through the Internet, comparing notes and discovering the good ideas of others. Thanks to this expanded ability to communicate, we know that many home remedies are sometimes just as effective as pharmaceuticals at treating the symptoms of minor ailments and even helping us to stay healthy and beautiful. . We also now have access to all the ingredients we need to keep our first aid kits and our kitchens stocked for any emergency.

Insect bites, bumps and bruises, headaches, and other minor ailments are often surprisingly easy to treat using simple home remedies. So are blemishes, cellulite, and other common beauty woes that affect nearly everyone at some time. Even your pets can benefit from simple home remedies for banishing fleas, eliminating dry, itchy skin, and treating a variety of other common issues.

The inexpensive remedies found in this book are very easy to make using a variety of ingredients, including simple food items and household products you probably have on hand right now. All ingredients, including the ones you'll need to shop for, are easy to find at supermarkets, drugstores, and health food stores. If you live in a rural area, you may find it easiest to obtain some items, such as essential oils, by shopping with an online retailer.

 Take Note Many pharmaceuticals began as home remedies. Quinine, for example, comes from the cinchona plant, which was used as a remedy for malaria. Aspirin emerged as a fever reducer found in wattle tree bark in South America and Africa.

What Are Home Remedies?

Just as the term suggests, home remedies are treatments that are known to provide simple pain relief or alleviate other symptoms by employing certain items that are easily procured; spices, fruits and vegetables, and even common household items can play important roles in home remedies.

While some home remedies don't always work well, countless others that have been shown to effectively treat minor ailments such as headaches, fevers, sprains and strains, and even the common cold. You might be surprised to discover that simple foods like honey, yogurt, and cinnamon are actually powerful healing agents with numerous uses.

You can probably think of some quick fixes for minor health problems; in fact, nearly everyone can recall certain remedies that have been passed down from one generation to the next. Though their origins have usually been forgotten, many simple pieces of advice passed down from great-great-grandparents live on. Whose idea was it to drink peppermint tea to soothe an aching stomach? Who figured out that oatmeal baths help ease itchy skin? No one can say for certain, but it's widely known that these simple home remedies work very well.

The simple at-home cures you'll find in this book work very well. All of them have passed the test of time. While some situations call for an intervention with modern medicine, many others do not. Home remedies help you feel better fast and can often help keep minor problems from worsening, so long as you intervene right away.

A Quick History of Home Remedies

For as long as humanity has been around, people have used foods and other substances to treat injuries and illnesses, often with surprising success. Archaeologists have shown that honey is among the oldest of all remedies still in use today; ancient Egyptians used it to reduce high blood pressure, and people today continue to use it to aid in healing wounds, alleviate athlete's foot, soothe burns, and treat a variety of other common problems.

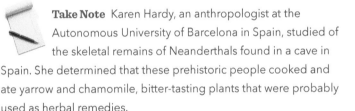

Take Note Karen Hardy, an anthropologist at the Autonomous University of Barcelona in Spain, studied of the skeletal remains of Neanderthals found in a cave in Spain. She determined that these prehistoric people cooked and ate yarrow and chamomile, bitter-tasting plants that were probably used as herbal remedies.

Ancient Assyrians used vinegar to treat earaches, and this popular home remedy was often used as a disinfectant and antiseptic before anyone knew about the connection between bacteria and infections. Today, science has proven that white vinegar and apple cider vinegar are useful for treating a wide array of maladies as well as for promoting general good health.

As time passed, medical knowledge grew and advances were made. During the Middle Ages, some treatments that did more harm than good, such as bloodletting and blistering became popular. Royalty and the rich were treated with therapies that included the application of scalding plasters made with pigeon dung and pitch, ingesting zinc sulfate and antimony, and inhaling pungent herbs meant to induce sneezing and eliminate "harmful humors." Not surprisingly, many of these patients died after being treated. Poorer citizens who fell ill and relied on old-fashioned remedies instead of doctors often regained their health—perhaps lucky that they couldn't afford expensive "cures." They went on to share the news with their neighbors about which home remedies worked best, and this knowledge continued to spread as everyday people used common ingredients to ease their symptoms.

As time passed, people continued to learn, through trial and error, how to heal themselves and their animal companions. Treatments that failed have been forgotten or relegated to books; those that worked well are in many cases used to this day.

Take Note Plant a garden and harvest your own home remedies. Dandelions help balance blood sugar, coneflower (Echinacea) can reduce the length of a cold, the scent of lavender relaxes you and soothes frayed nerves, and calendula can heal burned skin.

Most modern communities have plenty of thriving medical practices, but this hasn't always been the case. As recently as a century ago, people relied heavily on home remedies for treating all but the most serious of illnesses. Historical cookbooks contain many interesting recipes for treating a surprising number of common complaints, ranging from fever to dyspepsia. Some of the simplest old-fashioned treatments for indigestion, including eating raw carrot, fennel, or parsley, work very well and are still popular today.

Though quackery exists today, just as it has for millennia, popular home remedy treatments are often suitable alternatives for synthetic chemical products that actually contain the same healing compounds. For example, medicines made from plants rich in salicylates, which is the active ingredient in aspirin, were widely used throughout the ancient world. Egyptian papyri dating back to the second millennium BCE describe their use in pharmacology. Willow bark and willow bark extract were two popular sources of salicylates, and both have been noted for their effectiveness in treating pain, inflammation, and fever. Lewis and Clark are believed to have put willow bark tea to good use as they made their way across North America during their 1803–1806 expedition. Aspirin remains one of the world's most widely used medications, and is just one example of how manufacturers have modernized an ancient remedy and made it easily accessible to billions of people all over the planet.

While the Western world relies heavily on allopathic medicine, it is estimated that today about 50 percent of the world's population relies almost solely on folk medicine. Though some treatments have been proven to be ineffective, many others work very well and are gaining popularity, even in places where Western medicine is the standard.

Remedies from Around the World

Home remedies vary from one place to the next, and depend largely on the resources that are locally available, including foods, herbs and other plants, minerals, and essential oils.

Every remedy has a story and a place of origin. Allspice, for example, is useful for natural pain relief and as an antiseptic; it was first used in Central America. Bay leaves come from the Mediterranean bay laurel tree, and the medicines derived from these pungent leaves were first used by the Romans and Greeks.

Traditional Chinese medicine, which is based largely on the use of teas made from an array of natural ingredients, is the source of many popular home remedies. One example is the use of fresh or candied ginger for almost instant nausea relief. Another is to drink tea made with plenty of honey as an excellent way to eliminate constipation naturally.

Ayurveda, a form of natural medicine that originated in India, is another reliable source of home remedies that have gained popularity worldwide. Scientists now know that garlic and onions contain antibacterial compounds; Indian people have been using them for thousands of years to eliminate bacterial infections on the skin.

Take Note Many remedies involving essential oils, herbs, and other natural substances are now considered "complementary medicine" by the Western medical community. Your doctor may suggest one or more of the remedies listed in this book as part of your therapy for everything from a backache to cancer.

Like other indigenous peoples, Native Americans have extensive knowledge of the healing properties of natural ingredients, and have been passing natural remedies down from one generation to the next. Chamomile, milkweed, aloe, and dandelion are just a few of the plants Native American peoples have used to treat a wide array of symptoms, ranging from heartburn to fever. Echinacea, which is now widely taken for its ability to boost the immune system, is another popular home remedy that was first used by Native Americans.

These are just a few examples of home remedies from around the world. No matter where you go, you'll find that people use their own remedies quite effectively to treat common illnesses.

Frequently Asked Questions About Home Remedies

Q **What is the purpose of home remedies?**

Home remedies are intended to bring about effective relief from minor health problems in the simplest, least invasive way possible.

Q **Are home remedies expensive?**

Quite the opposite. Almost all home remedies are surprisingly inexpensive. A few items, such as pure essential oils, are more expensive, but you use them in small quantities, so a little will go a long way.

Q **I take prescription medication. Can I still use home remedies?**

If you take prescription drugs, you should discuss with your health-care provider any home remedies you are considering. Some remedies can cause adverse drug reactions, while others can reduce the potency of prescriptions. Never assume that a remedy is not potent simply because it is natural.

Q **I have leftover prescription drugs on hand. Can I use those as home remedies?**

No. Prescription drugs are safe only for the person they were written for, at the time they were written. Sometimes, a new problem seems just like an old problem, but in fact, you need a different medication—or perhaps you don't need a prescription at all. If you have old prescriptions, discuss your current problem with a medical professional to determine whether it is advisable to use them in your current circumstances. And even if you have the right drug, the medication may have passed its expiration date, so be sure to check. Old prescriptions should not be discarded by flushing them down the toilet, because they can get into the water system—even if you have a septic tank. Drop off your old prescriptions at any pharmacy for disposal.

Q **Will what I eat make a difference in ensuring the remedies I use are able to work correctly?**

Dietary habits affect all aspects of life; when you eat properly, your body is well nourished at a cellular level, creating an internal environment that is conducive to healing. Following a well-balanced diet is never a bad idea.

Q **Are home remedies safe for children?**

While many home remedies are safe for children, others are too potent for them to take safely, and some topical preparations might be too strong for a young child's tender skin. If you are considering using home remedies to treat a child, check with a health professional to ensure they are safe for children before use.

Q **I have strange symptoms and am not sure what's wrong with me. Should I use home remedies to try to clear them up?**

If you're not certain what the problem is, it is safer to go to the doctor for a correct diagnosis before using any home remedies. Failing to get *an accurate diagnosis could make the problem worse, as could treating it incorrectly.*

Q Do home remedies have any side effects?

Most home remedies have no side effects. The ones found in this book have been carefully selected for their safety and reliability. If you notice any undesirable side effects, stop the treatment immediately.

Q I have the ingredients on hand for a remedy I want to try, but they are expired. What should I do?

If items you have on hand are out of date, buy new ingredients. These remedies work best when ingredients are freshest, as that is when they are most potent.

Q What will happen if I mistakenly take the wrong remedy?

Since the remedies in this book use everyday foods and household items, they are extremely safe. You should suffer no ill effects if you take an incorrect remedy by mistake, but your problem isn't likely to go away. Use the proper remedy as soon as you discover that you've made an error.

Q Is it possible to overdose on home remedies?

While the potential for overdose is extremely slim, always use the right amount of the remedy you've selected. Using more or less may not give you the desired effect. If you are allergic or sensitive to an ingredient in a home remedy, do not use that remedy, because it is likely to do more harm than good. For some remedies, though, such as drinking lots of fluids when suffering from a cold or the flu, you need to do it continuously. If this is the case, it will be noted in the treatment's instructions.

Q I made more of a particular remedy than I can use right away. Is there a way to save it?

Many remedies can be stored in a cool, dark place inside a sealed glass container for as long as three weeks. However, many remedies are most potent right after they have been made, so you're probably better off making only what you can use right away. If you like, you can pre-measure the ingredients and store them in separate containers, and then mix them together when you are ready to use them. This is convenient and will ensure that your preparations are potent. Be sure to date items you prepackage to ensure they are not expired when you finally use them.

Q Can I grow my own herbs for use in home remedies?

Yes. In fact, you may be better off growing your own herbs organically. You'll save money and have fresh herbs on hand any time you need them. As an added bonus, many of the best medicinal herbs are also fantastic for culinary use.

Q Some of the home remedies I've heard about seem a little odd. Should I try them anyway?

As long as a treatment you hear about doesn't sound like it will harm you, consider trying it. The home remedies in this book are all effective; even if they sound strange, they're worth trying. This being said, there are many strange remedies that probably won't work—sleeping with a bar of soap in your bed to alleviate leg cramps is just one of many ineffective so-called remedies.

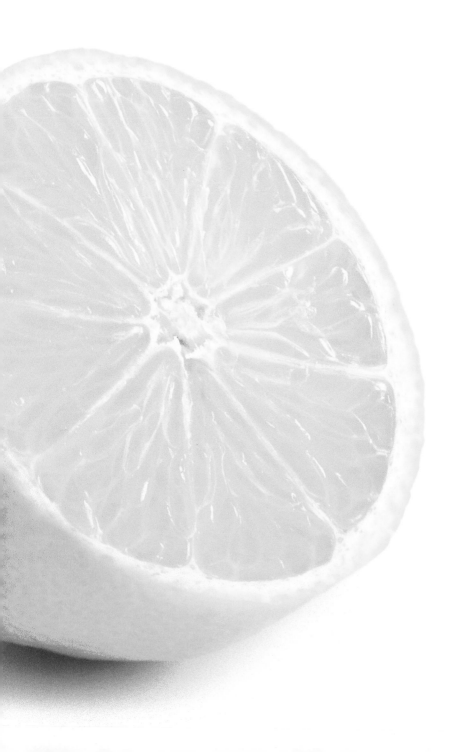

CHAPTER 2

Getting Started with Home Remedies

Most home remedies are wonderfully simple, and many of them use items that are commonly found in most households. Baking soda, vinegar, lemons, herbal tea, and table salt are just a few of the many items you can use to speed healing and promote overall health. A tea kettle or saucepan for boiling water, a spoon for stirring, and a teacup or water glass are some of the simple tools you can use to treat mild health problems ranging from hiccups to a sore throat.

Keep basic first aid supplies on hand, both at home and in your vehicle. If you enjoy camping, backpacking, or other outdoor activities, make simple first aid kits to keep with you during your adventures, as well. This way, you'll never be far from your favorite remedies. Besides bandages, cotton swabs, and other standard first aid supplies, pack items you think you may need for treating the problems that are most likely to occur in certain situations. If, for example, you often suffer from carsickness or seasickness, pack candied ginger or strong natural ginger candies so you can take ginger when motion sickness spoils your fun. Be creative as you create your own first aid kits and you'll always be prepared for nearly any challenge that comes your way. (For more advice about putting together a first aid kit, see the Appendix.)

How to Use Home Remedies

Each of the remedies presented in this book is accompanied by precise instructions for its use. Following these instructions will increase the likelihood that the remedy you use will be effective.

Remedies are administered in a variety of ways. Some are taken orally, while others are used topically. Some are very simple to prepare, but others call for precise formulation. Read through the instructions before beginning any remedy, so that you know what is expected.

Why use a remedy topically instead of orally? In many cases, a topical solution only works if applied directly to an affected area. In most cases, ingesting a topical solution would also be dangerous. Topical creams, lotions, ointments, and gels are used for afflictions on the skin, while eye drops and asthma inhalants—also considered topical remedies—are most effective when applied directly to the membrane. Oral remedies often need to metabolize throughout the body to work, or they need to reach a specific internal organ. For example, ginger tea won't help your stomach distress if you rub it on your tummy; it needs to be inside your stomach to work. An ointment with a eucalyptus or menthol component, however, will relieve congestion in your bronchial passages if rubbed on your chest.

Many common symptoms can be treated with a variety of different remedies. Use just one treatment at a time so that it has an opportunity to do its work. While some simple remedies act rapidly to provide almost instant relief, others take longer.

It's important to remember that many common illnesses, such as the cold and flu, are caused by viruses that can be spread by simple contact. The remedies recommended are intended to treat your symptoms and make you feel more comfortable, and although they may shorten the duration or severity of your illness, they don't kill viruses. If you are sick, limit your contact with others. Wash your hands frequently and use disinfectant spray on phones, door handles, remote controls, light switches, and other items that others touch or use. This can help to prevent sickness from spreading.

Take Note virus invades your cells and multiplies inside your body. With rare exceptions, a virus cannot be treated with drugs and simply must run its course. Bacteria, on the other hand, can be killed by antibiotics. The fastest way to get over a bacterial infection (strep throat, tuberculosis, pneumonia) is to see your doctor for a prescription.

Finally, remember to keep yourself well hydrated at all times, and even more so when you're not feeling well. By staying properly hydrated, you ensure that healing agents, including vitamins, minerals, and other nutrients, are able to make their way throughout your body and work more effectively. Just staying hydrated can help minimize symptoms such as a sore throat and headache. Drink lots of water and caffeine-free tea to help keep your system working as efficiently as possible.

Take Note Focus on keeping the whole body healthy. Often, sickness seems to affect certain functions or body parts, and there's a tendency to focus on those symptoms while neglecting the rest of the body. Treat yourself to special care, particularly when you are not feeling your best. Taking a warm bath or hot shower, using a natural moisturizing lotion, and cuddling up with a favorite book or movie can be wonderfully restful. Staying calm, avoiding stressful situations, and just resting quietly are some good ways to stay balanced while your body does its healing work.

When to Use Home Remedies

You can try a home remedy any time you are experiencing symptoms you recognize. For example, if you have clogged sinuses, a runny nose, a mild sore throat, a low fever, minor muscle pain, and a headache, you probably have a cold or the flu. All these symptoms can be alleviated with simple home remedies, which are gentler than over-the-counter medications. In many cases, the recommended remedies, such as drinking hot tea, help support the body so it can work its hardest to fight off a viral infection. At the same time, drinking liquids helps promote hydration, which in turn helps alleviate headaches—and that alone helps you feel much better. Warm liquids also thin mucous and soothe your throat while providing a feeling of overall comfort—something cold medicine doesn't really do.

Home remedies are intended to provide relief of mild symptoms and are not a substitute for professional medical care. Use home remedies only if you are absolutely certain that the symptoms you are experiencing are associated with a specific ailment.

These remedies are often excellent for first aid, and in many cases a simple treatment is all you will need. If you need quick pain relief from a bug bite or bee sting, a home remedy is likely to do the trick. If you've got an upset stomach, motion sickness, or heartburn, there are myriad easy ways to alleviate the discomfort with one of the many tried and true remedies you'll soon become familiar with.

If a home remedy does not seem to be working, you may want to try another remedy. If the problem gets worse, seek medical attention. The last thing you want to do is to allow a problem to become serious. There's always the possibility that an underlying health problem is causing symptoms to pop up, and if that's the case, home remedies need to be set aside in favor of professional treatment.

 Take Note Use home remedies to enhance wellness. Boost your immune system with a diet that includes vegetables and fruits of many colors, nuts, berries, dark chocolate, fish, yogurt, garlic, tea, sweet potatoes, and mushrooms—all foods that contain important vitamins that fight off infection and viruses.

When Not to Use Home Remedies

While simple home remedies can be effective in many cases, there are times when it's best not to try treating ailments or injuries on your own. See a medical professional if your symptoms are acute or unusual. Seek emergency medical treatment for serious sprains and suspected fractures. You can use home remedies to treat minor burns, but large burns or those involving blisters or open skin are serious and need to be treated by a medical professional.

If you have tried a home remedy for any type of injury or illness and the condition worsens instead of improving, consult your doctor. In addition, do not use home remedies to try to alleviate chest pain, and if you are having difficulty breathing, get to the doctor.

A high or persistent fever is often a symptom of a serious problem, so don't take chances; see the doctor. You should also see the doctor if severe vomiting and diarrhea are part of your illness. Though these symptoms often go away on their own and can respond well to home remedies, they can cause rapid debilitation when severe. If the treatments you are trying are not working, call your doctor.

If you have cold symptoms that just won't go away, such as severe throat pain, persistent headaches, and constant congestion, you could be suffering from an infection, in which case you will need to see the doctor, possibly for antibiotics. If you suspect you have any kind of infection, seek treatment before it worsens and spreads. This can happen rapidly and can ultimately lead to death, so don't wait for treatment.

Finally, home remedies are not intended to replace drug therapy and other treatments prescribed by your doctor. If you'd like to use a certain remedy in conjunction with a prescription or other treatment, talk to your health-care provider before using even the simplest of at-home cures. This is particularly true if you are being treated for a serious illness such as cancer, lung disease, or heart disease. Drug interactions can cause your condition to worsen, and they can lead to death.

When to Seek Medical Attention

Even though home remedies are often effective, there are times when it's best to get medical help right away to prevent the injury or illness from becoming worse, and to rule out serious conditions that could be life-threatening. Some of these situations are:

- Animal bites with punctured skin
- Back pain beyond occasional stiffness or soreness
- Blackouts
- Bladder pain
- Chest pain
- Difficulty breathing
- Eye injury or suspected eye infection
- Frequent headaches
- Head and neck injuries
- Inability to bear weight or pressure on an injured limb or joint
- Infections of any type, including boils and abscesses
- Kidney pain
- Painful, throbbing feet and legs
- Pain, redness, and swelling that doesn't respond to initial treatment
- Scabs, sores, or rashes that don't respond to initial treatment
- Serious bleeding
- Serious joint injuries, including dislocation
- Serious skin conditions, such as suspected ringworm, scabies, or impetigo
- Serious swelling around a bee sting site (possible allergic reaction)
- Severe abdominal pain with fever
- Snakebite
- Suspected ear infection
- Suspected fracture
- Suspected sexually transmitted diseases, such as HPV
- Suspected urinary tract infection
- Swollen lymph nodes
- Swollen or lumpy testicles
- Yellowish skin or whites of eyes (possible jaundice)

Take Note If you are treating a child with a home remedy and you don't see the results you want after the expected course of the treatment or within a few minutes for more serious ailments and symptoms, it's always the best course to call your pediatrician—especially if your child has a fever above 102 degrees Fahrenheit, is in pain, or has trouble breathing. If the child is having an asthmatic attack, a severe allergic reaction, or anaphylaxis, skip the home remedy and go straight to the nearest emergency room.

Tips and Techniques for Using Home Remedies

Home remedies are often quick and simple to use. Begin each treatment by ensuring you have all the necessary ingredients and supplies on hand. Set up everything you will need for your treatment, considering each step carefully. Only when you feel you are familiar with the necessary steps should you begin the treatment.

Many treatments are meant to alleviate the discomfort caused by physical symptoms, so they may need to be repeated, depending on how you feel. If, for example, you have a cold and are treating your sore throat and stuffy sinuses by drinking hot liquids, you can simply keep drinking those liquids as often as you like so that you are as comfortable as possible.

No matter which treatment or treatments you are using, be sure to follow instructions carefully, and do not skip any steps. Though relief often comes very quickly, there are times when your symptoms will disappear slowly. For instance, if you're suffering from a headache and are using a home remedy to get rid of it, your head pain isn't likely to disappear immediately. Be patient, relax, and wait for the recommended amount of time. If you are still uncomfortable and want to try another remedy, you can do so then.

Take Note Be wary of the new "miracle" remedies that pop up on the Internet on a regular basis. All too often, their claims of overnight cures, huge health benefits (especially weight loss or restoration of youth), and simplicity are marketing schemes for a specific pill—usually one that's completely untested.

If certain health problems seem to occur frequently, pay attention to what's happening before those problems start. If, for example, you suffer regularly from an upset stomach and heartburn, think about your diet and other factors that affect your digestion, and start taking preventive action. Often, greasy or spicy foods are followed by queasiness. Sometimes the culprit is stress. Eliminate potential causes one by one, paying careful attention to the way you feel afterward. Eliminating the problem by preventing it is easier than taking even the simplest of remedies.

Finally, never hesitate to seek medical attention if you feel it is warranted, particularly if you seem to suffer from the same symptoms over and over. If you have tried a few home remedies and they're not working, make an appointment with your doctor. If you are suffering from one of the serious or potentially life-threatening conditions listed earlier in this chapter, the best course of action is to immediately seek emergency medical treatment.

PART II

HANDY HEALERS

3 Healing Foods

4 Healing Household Products

5 Healing Essential Oils

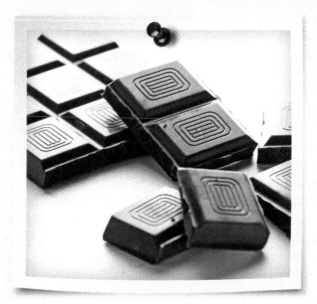

HEALING FOODS

- Apples
- Bananas
- Celery
- Cinnamon
- Cranberries
- Dark
  Chocolate
- Flaxseed
- Garlic
- Ginger
- Honey
- Kale
- Lemons
- Mushrooms
- Nuts
- Oats
- Papayas
- Peppermint
- Pineapple
- Red Wine
- Yogurt

CHAPTER 3

Healing Foods

The ancient Greek mathematician, astronomer, and physician Hippocrates once said, "Let food be thy medicine and medicine be thy food." We are constantly bombarded with information about how to eat right, yet many of us suffer from chronic diseases, including those related to obesity. In part, this is due to an unhealthful tendency to rely on packaged and fast foods that taste fantastic but do nothing to promote health. These foods are tempting because they're easy to find and equally easy to prepare; in fact, many require no preparation at all. But this is not the way our bodies were designed to eat.

Eliminating packaged and fast foods from our diets in favor of a wide variety of whole, natural foods is an excellent way to improve overall health. Many foods also specifically promote healing. Not only do these foods provide the body with important nutrients, they are delicious and satisfying, too.

Many healing foods can be either eaten or applied topically. Several contain potent antioxidants, enzymes, and flavonoids, while others contain specific compounds that aid in promoting health and healing. Whether you are hoping to improve your immunity, fight a cold or other virus, or soothe a sunburn or other skin irritation, these foods can help.

Apples

Apples are highly nutritious and low in calories, with an abundance of soluble and insoluble fiber, plus vitamins, minerals, and antioxidants. They contain high levels of quercetin (a flavonoid that promotes heart health), and apples are among the few sources of the flavonoid phloridzin (which is good for your bones).

BENEFITS

People who eat apples regularly benefit in a number of ways. Quercetin is linked to improved heart and vascular health, and has been shown to help inhibit the growth of breast, colon, lung, and prostate cancer cells. It is also an effective histamine blocker that helps ease inflammation caused by allergies. It also aids in the production of fibronectin and collagen, two substances that are necessary for healthy skin and joints.

Phloridzin (sometimes referred to as phlorizin) has been shown to reduce the risk of osteoporosis and may even help increase bone density. The high levels of pectin in apples aid in reducing LDL (bad) cholesterol.

The soluble fiber in apples has also been shown to help keep blood sugar levels stable and sweep blood vessels clean. The high levels of insoluble fiber in apples make them an ideal food for good digestion as well as for weight management.

HOW TO USE

Apples are best consumed raw, with the skin intact. You can juice them, add them to smoothies, put them in salads, and crunch on them any time you are craving a snack. If you hope to benefit from phloridzin, be sure not to peel yours. You can also purchase the extract and take it as directed.

TIPS AND PRECAUTIONS

Many of the vital nutrients apples contain are located in or just beneath the skin. Buy organic apples to reduce your exposure to pesticides, and be sure to make or buy a produce wash so you can clean your fruits and vegetables thoroughly before consuming them.

Eat at least one apple a day to enjoy as many benefits as possible, but eat your apple with or after a meal, rather than on its own. A study published in the *Journal of Dentistry* in 2011 showed that people who ate apples were almost four times more likely to have dental damage than people who did not. This effect was mitigated if the apples were eaten with meals, and increased if the apples were eaten on their own in the middle of the day.

Apple seeds contain cyanide, a naturally occurring and powerful poison. You would need to eat an awful lot of apple seeds to feel the poison's effects, but there's no reason to tempt fate. Avoid eating the seeds as best you can.

Bananas

A favorite with people of all ages, bananas are sweet, filling, and easy to carry and consume. They are high in potassium, fiber, tryptophan, vitamin A, and iron, along with many other essential vitamins and minerals.

BENEFITS

The potassium bananas contain makes them a good choice for promoting circulatory health, and their carbohydrates make them an excellent food for fast, steady energy that will keep you going for hours.

The fiber in bananas is structured in a way that makes them perfect for restoring and maintaining regular bowel function. Those who suffer from constipation find bananas help relieve it; those suffering from diarrhea find that eating bananas along with rice, applesauce, and toast (the BRAT diet) helps relieve that problem, too. The BRAT diet is also a good choice for anyone suffering from gastrointestinal distress. As it is not nutritionally complete, this plan should be followed for just a day or two, until digestive balance is restored. Other foods can be added as tolerated—some to try include plain skinless chicken, yogurt, and tapioca.

The tryptophan and vitamin B$_6$ bananas contain can help elevate your spirits when you're feeling a little moody or depressed, and they can also help alleviate cravings associated with nicotine withdrawal.

HOW TO USE

Bananas are wonderful eaten on their own, and they're also ideal for adding to smoothies. They can be mashed and added to baked goods such as muffins and quick breads, where they can be used to replace some of the fat in recipes while adding moisture and natural sweetness.

TIPS AND PRECAUTIONS

Bananas need to ripen out of the refrigerator, ideally hanging on a hook. If you have bananas that are in danger of becoming overripe and you cannot use them immediately, peel them, cut them in chunks, and store them in the freezer for later use in smoothies and baked goods.

It is actually possible to eat too many bananas. The vasodilators in bananas can cause headaches, and for some people they can be a migraine trigger. Tryptophan is a natural sedative, and the amino acids in bananas can block amino acids from entering your brain and keeping you alert—so eating several bananas can make you sleepy. Eating up to a dozen can create an excess of potassium in your system, which can cause nausea and an irregular heartbeat, or even cardiac arrest. However, one to two bananas a day can provide a good balance of nutrients.

Celery

Celery is very high in folic acid, potassium, B vitamins, calcium, vitamin C, and fiber. It contains a number of other important nutrients, yet it is extremely low in calories, so it's a great choice to add to recipes of all kinds.

BENEFITS

Celery isn't just good for you, it's also a wonderful home remedy for fighting bad breath. The rough, insoluble fiber it contains helps scrub plaque from teeth and remove food particles from the tongue. Munch on a celery stick after eating, and you'll notice that your breath stays fresh longer. Celery and celery seed are also natural painkillers. If you suffer from gout, try eating four stalks of celery daily. If you don't like the idea of chewing all that celery, you can juice it or, unless you are pregnant, breastfeeding, or allergic to celery, take celery seed extract.

Why It Works Celery contains high levels of COX-2 inhibitors, a form of nonsteroidal anti-inflammatory drug (NSAID). Celery seed extract helps alleviate minor aches without the side effects of over-the-counter drugs. Gout sufferers benefit from celery's COX-2 inhibitors because the compound helps reduce high uric-acid levels that lead to gout attacks.

HOW TO USE

The root, stalks, leaves, and seeds of the celery plant are edible, but the stalks and leaves are easiest to find in stores. You can simply munch on celery stalks plain, top them with a little nut butter or soft cheese, or cut them up and add them to soups, stews, salads, and other foods. Celery is an excellent addition to stir-fries and other dishes, too.

TIPS AND PRECAUTIONS

Raw celery is best for you, so if you're hoping to enjoy as many of the benefits of celery as you can, try to eat most of your celery without cooking it first. Celery should be washed very well before being eaten, and since conventionally grown celery is often heavily doused with pesticides, it's best to purchase organic if possible.

While the science has not been conclusive, celery oil and celery seeds are not recommended for women who are pregnant or breastfeeding.

Large amounts of celery might cause the uterus to contract, which could lead to a miscarriage. Celery eaten as part of a meal is safe, but extracts and concentrations may be dangerous.

It's hard to imagine that a food as innocuous as celery could cause an allergic reaction, but people who are sensitive to a complex of related plants—wild carrot, mugwort, birch, and dandelion—may also be allergic to celery.

Cinnamon

Cinnamon has a sweet scent and a warm, pleasant flavor that makes it a favorite with cooks and bakers all over the world. This simple spice is high in manganese, iron, fiber, and calcium.

BENEFITS

Cinnamon contains several beneficial compounds, which is why it has a long history of use in traditional medicine. If you have high cholesterol, taking as little as ½ teaspoon of cinnamon daily may help lower LDL (bad) cholesterol levels. It can also help keep blood sugar levels stable, and studies have shown that it may be useful in regulating type 2 diabetes.

This sweet, delicious spice is also an excellent natural appetite suppressant. When eaten with regular meals, it helps keep you feeling satisfied so you're less likely to reach for snacks later in the day.

HOW TO USE

Powdered cinnamon is very easy to add to dishes of all kinds. It tends to float on top of liquids, so you'll find that it's best to blend it with other ingredients before adding it to recipes. If you're making a smoothie, for example, dust the fruit with cinnamon before putting the fruit in the blender, and you'll find the cinnamon is much easier to incorporate.

Make sure you are buying real cinnamon and not a similar-smelling spice called cassia. True cinnamon costs a little more than cassia, but cassia offers none of the benefits cinnamon does. In addition, high doses of cassia cinnamon may be toxic, especially if you have liver problems.

If you are hoping to stabilize your blood sugar using cinnamon, do not discontinue any of your prescribed medications. You will need to continue working with your doctor to ensure that cinnamon and any other dietary and/or lifestyle changes you are making are having the desired effect.

Cinnamon in the quantities found in foods is safe for anyone, but high doses are not recommended for pregnant or breastfeeding women or for children. The possibility of liver issues and cinnamon's ability to lower blood sugar can be harmful during pregnancy or to young children.

Cranberries

One cup of cranberries contains just forty-five calories, but they are loaded with antioxidants. These tart red berries also contain high levels of vitamins, minerals, and fiber.

BENEFITS

Cranberries are highly acidic and help keep the urinary tract clear of bacteria that can lead to painful infections. They are also excellent for heart and vascular health, and studies have shown that compounds they contain have the ability to inhibit the growth of skin, prostate, brain, and lung cancer cells.

Why It Works Cranberries contain compounds called proanthocyanidins, or condensed tannins, that keep bacteria from adhering to the inside of the urinary tract. This allows the bladder to flush out any bacteria along with the cranberry juice.

HOW TO USE

You'll gain the greatest benefits from cranberries by consuming the whole fruit rather than the juice alone. If you do drink cranberry juice, opt for 100 percent juice without added sugar or artificial sweeteners. Dried cranberries can be added to cereal, and whole fresh cranberries are great in smoothies and other foods. Cranberry supplements in powdered or pill form are also an excellent option for anyone who wants to enjoy the benefits these powerful berries offer.

TIPS AND PRECAUTIONS

Although cranberries are good for digestion and can help prevent ulcers, eating too many of them can contribute to gastrointestinal distress. If large amounts of fruit tend to give you diarrhea, try cranberry supplements.

Some people are allergic to cranberries, and those who take antacids, blood thinners, and anti-alcohol prescriptions such as Antabuse can suffer from adverse side effects from cranberry supplements. If in doubt, talk to your doctor before adding cranberries to your daily diet.

Take Note Antioxidants are important to counteract the effects of free radicals. The body generates free radicals as part of the process of converting food into energy. Free radicals can also be found in the air and in reactions in the skin caused by exposure to sunlight. They harm the body by stealing electrons from cells, which changes the cells' structure or function. Antioxidants counteract this effect by giving electrons to free radicals.

Dark Chocolate

Dark chocolate has an irresistible flavor, which it gets from the cocoa solids it contains. Dark chocolate is chocolate without any added milk solids. It has a more chocolaty taste than milk chocolate. It is also high in vitamins, minerals, and antioxidants, and it contains several beneficial compounds, including catechins, flavonoids, theobromine, and phenylethylamine.

BENEFITS

Chocolate is often seen as a decadent treat, but when not overly processed, it offers many outstanding health benefits and can be used to promote wellness. Dark chocolate has been linked with healthful blood pressure levels as well as with reduced risk of heart attack and stroke. In addition, the antioxidants it contains have been found to contribute to cardiovascular health.

Dark chocolate also increases the brain's serotonin level. Because of this, it is an excellent remedy for alleviating PMS symptoms.

Why It Works Dark chocolate contains theobromine, a mild stimulant. While this energy boost alone might leave you feeling good, the phenylethylamine in dark chocolate is also a mild stimulant as well as an antidepressant. An ounce or two of dark chocolate can put you in a better mood almost instantly.

HOW TO USE

The best and fastest way to enjoy dark chocolate is to eat it. Unwrap it, savor the aroma, take a small bite, and allow it to melt on your tongue. Swallow it and repeat.

A small amount of dark chocolate is much more satisfying than larger amounts of milk chocolate or white chocolate. The higher the cacao content, the less you'll need to feel better.

TIPS AND PRECAUTIONS

If you're not used to the flavor of dark chocolate, you may find it to be overly intense at first. Gradually accustom yourself to darker and darker chocolate, and soon you'll be a connoisseur of the darkest varieties available.

If you are prone to migraines, dark chocolate can be a trigger. Test yourself with a small amount. If you suffer from a migraine after eating dark chocolate, this healing food is one that's best left off your menu.

Flaxseed

Flaxseeds might be tiny, but they are packed with nutrients, including omega-3 fatty acids, fiber, and lignans, which are chemical compounds with antioxidant properties. Flaxseed has a pleasant, nutty flavor.

BENEFITS

Beyond promoting good health, when consumed regularly flaxseed can help alleviate a number of inflammatory conditions. These include allergies, asthma, and arthritis. Studies have suggested that flaxseed also helps to reduce inflammation associated with a buildup of arterial plaque, thus aiding in the prevention of stroke and heart attack.

The lignans in flaxseed help keep hormone levels balanced and can even offer some protection against cancers that are linked to hormone levels, including breast cancer, colon cancer, and prostate cancer. They may also aid in promoting cardiovascular health and preventing osteoporosis. Eating four tablespoons of ground flaxseed daily may help reduce LDL (bad) cholesterol.

HOW TO USE

Though flaxseed can be eaten whole, most of the nutrients are locked inside the tiny seeds and are only accessible to the body when the seeds are ground or soaked before being added to smoothies. You can either purchase ground flaxseed or grind it yourself.

Sprinkle ground flaxseed on cereal, mix it into baked goods, stir it into soups and stews, and use it to top your morning yogurt.

Flax oil does have some benefits, but it does not contain all the components found in whole ground flaxseed. Since these components work together to produce the desired effects, it's best to consume ground flax-seed rather than flaxseed oil.

TIPS AND PRECAUTIONS

Like other fresh foods, flaxseed is prone to spoilage. Buy only as much as you can reasonably use within a month, and store it in the refrigerator.

Since flaxseed can affect estrogen levels, you should not supplement your diet with flaxseed if you are pregnant or nursing.

The Mayo Clinic notes that flaxseed may lower blood pressure and blood sugar levels. If you are already taking medications for these conditions, let your doctor know that you have added flaxseed to your diet so you can monitor your levels together.

It's important to take in ten times as much liquid as the amount of flax-seed you eat to avoid bowel obstructions and other digestive issues. This may sound daunting, but think of it as ten tablespoons (five ounces) of water for every tablespoon of flaxseed you consume.

Take Note Omega-3 fatty acids are essential for many normal body functions, including controlling blood clotting and building cell membranes in the brain. They are also associated with many health benefits, including protection against heart disease and possibly even stroke. New studies suggest potential benefits for a wide range of conditions, including cancer, inflammatory bowel disease, and other autoimmune diseases. We cannot synthesize omega-3s in the body, so we must get them from our diet.

Garlic

Garlic is very high in minerals, including magnesium, calcium, selenium, and manganese, and it is an excellent source of many vitamins, antioxidants, and phytonutrients. It also contains thiosulfinate compounds (which help lower cholesterol levels) and important enzymes.

BENEFITS

A very popular ingredient in a variety of foods, garlic is known for its many health benefits. One of its thiosulfinate compounds is credited with increasing vascular health and reducing the risk of both stroke and coronary artery disease. This same compound gives garlic its antiviral, antifungal, and antibacterial properties, which, along with its vitamin and mineral content, make it an excellent choice any time you are suffering from a cold or the flu.

Garlic oil has long been used as an effective treatment for fungal infections, including ringworm, and raw chopped garlic is traditionally used as a remedy for skin problems, including topical yeast infections.

Why It Works Garlic produces a compound called allicin, which gives it its pungent odor. Scientists have discovered that this compound has the ability to battle microbes, including the bacteria that create MRSA, a staph infection found primarily in hospitals. Garlic also appears to be effective in combating herpes simplex virus type 1 and 2, influenza B, and a number of other viruses. Studies so far are too small to be considered conclusive, but the results are promising.

HOW TO USE

Many people enjoy the taste of garlic in recipes, but raw garlic is an acquired taste. Luckily, if you dislike the flavor of garlic but want to enjoy the many health benefits it offers, you can take it in tablet or capsule form.

TIPS AND PRECAUTIONS

If you eat a lot of garlic, you may start smelling garlicky. This is because the plant's sulfide compounds are excreted in the body's sweat. If this becomes a problem, take odorless garlic tablets to keep your consumption level up and eliminate associated body odor and halitosis.

When crushed, thiosulfinate compounds form allicin, which acts as a blood thinner, so anyone taking anticoagulants such as warfarin should avoid excessive consumption. If you take blood thinners, talk to your doctor before increasing your garlic intake.

Ginger

Ginger contains an anti-inflammatory compound called gingerol along with volatile oils called shogaol and zingerone that give it its characteristic spicy fragrance and sweet aroma. The rhizome also has as much as 3 percent essential oil, which contains compounds called sesquiterpenoids that may potentially be helpful in preventing cardiovascular disease and cancer.

BENEFITS

The benefits of ginger are numerous. It is an excellent remedy for nausea and vomiting brought on by illness or motion sickness. Tea made with fresh ginger is an excellent remedy for congestion associated with allergies or the common cold. It can also ease sore throats and calm coughs. Ginger tea is also an effective headache remedy that can sometimes alleviate pain associated with migraines.

Ginger tea and foods containing plenty of fresh ginger have been shown to be effective in easing minor body pain. When applied topically, ginger can ease the pain of joint injuries, muscle injuries, arthritis, and rheumatism. A paste made with fresh ginger can help to alleviate minor dental pain.

Cancer researchers have found that ginger may be an effective agent against ovarian cancer and in providing protection from colon cancer. Studies have shown that ginger may also decrease tumor formation in people who have been exposed to chemicals linked to the formation of cancerous cells. While it isn't wise to forgo medical treatment or routine tests, ginger can be a valuable addition to your anti-cancer arsenal.

HOW TO USE

While powdered ginger is usually used in baked goods, fresh ginger contains the highest levels of gingerol and other substances associated with ginger's healing powers. To make ginger tea, buy fresh ginger root, peel it, and slice it thinly or grate it before steeping it in boiling water until the tea is cool enough to drink. Sweeten your tea with local honey to make it even better for you.

Fresh ginger is also a great addition to stir-fries, curries, and other dishes. It is usually thinly sliced or finely chopped before being added to recipes. Like other pungent spices, a little goes a long way.

You can also enjoy fresh ginger in smoothies and juices. Be sure to peel it before adding it to your blender or juicer. It pairs well with fruits such as apples, bananas, and pears.

TIPS AND PRECAUTIONS

Powdered ginger is fine for baking, but don't try to consume it in place of fresh ginger, as its possible side effects include bloating, gas, nausea, and heartburn—some symptoms, oddly enough, that fresh ginger can alleviate.

Ginger promotes the production of bile and can cause people with gallstones to suffer worse symptoms. It also interacts with blood thinners, including warfarin, and may increase the risk of bruising or bleeding. When taken in large amounts, ginger can lower blood sugar, which may increase the risk of hypoglycemia. If you take prescription drugs for high blood pressure, ginger may lower your blood pressure farther than desired, or it may cause an irregular heartbeat. Talk with your doctor before adding high-dose ginger to your diet.

Honey

Honey is a naturally sweet food produced by honeybees using nectar collected from flowers. It gets its sweetness from glucose and fructose, and it also contains enzymes, vitamins, and minerals. It ranges in color from nearly clear to dark amber, depending on what flowers the bees used to produce it.

BENEFITS

The benefits of honey are many. It provides quick energy for superior athletic performance and reduced muscle fatigue, and that's just the beginning. Raw honey from your local area, which contains a small amount of pollen, can help alleviate allergy symptoms by building up your tolerance to local pollens. In addition, it has antibacterial and antioxidant properties that can help improve your overall health. Researchers have also found that people who consume raw honey regularly are less susceptible to cancer than those who do not.

Honey's antibacterial properties make it an excellent home remedy for treating numerous skin problems, including yeast infections and athlete's foot. It may be applied to minor wounds and minor burns to speed healing and reduce the potential for scarring.

Because of its ability to soothe inflammation, honey is an excellent home remedy for sore throats and coughs. When added to tea made with fresh lemon juice, it helps alleviate the discomfort caused by congestion associated with allergies and colds.

Why It Works Glucose and fructose in honey metabolize as sugar does, providing a burst of energy. Pollen in local honey may help you build a tolerance to pollens that cause allergies. Honey over a wound seals in moisture, which is important for healing. This protective barrier and honey's antibacterial properties inhibits infection.

HOW TO USE

Purchase local honey and store it at room temperature so it doesn't crystallize. If your honey does crystallize, you can place the jar in a pan of very hot water. Allow it to sit for ten to fifteen minutes, or until the honey has liquefied.

TIPS AND PRECAUTIONS

Raw honey is best for use in home remedies, because it contains enzymes and pollen. Pasteurized honey tastes nice but is not nearly as potent.

Do not give honey to infants younger than eighteen months old. It contains low levels of botulinum spores, which occur naturally but can cause serious illness and even death in babies, who have immature digestive systems incapable of processing the substance. Infants should not be given products that contain honey, even in small amounts—crackers, cereals, and other processed foods that contain it have the potential to cause serious illness or death.

Many women are concerned about whether honey is safe when they are pregnant or breastfeeding. Since an adult's digestive system processes the botulinum spores in honey completely, it is safe for pregnant and nursing women to consume—in fact, it can help ease morning sickness and heartburn associated with pregnancy.

Kale

Kale is a dark, leafy green vegetable belonging to the cabbage family that is extremely high in vitamins, minerals, and antioxidants. It also contains high levels of sulforaphane (a molecule with antimicrobial properties), indoles (the parent molecule for serotonin and other compounds), and vitamins, including 1,328 percent of the recommended daily allowance of vitamin K per cup. It is also an excellent source of iron, calcium, and vitamins A and C.

BENEFITS

The sulforaphane in kale contains is a powerful compound that helps guard against breast, gastric, prostate, and skin cancers. The indoles it contains have also been found to be effective in protecting against breast cancer as well as colon, and cervical cancers, and the high levels of vitamin K help build strong bones, promote healthful blood clotting, and prevent heart disease.

Because of its high nutrient content, kale is an excellent home remedy for cold prevention. When enjoyed regularly, it can help promote healthy, younger-looking skin.

HOW TO USE

Kale is wonderful in salads. It may also be sautéed or boiled, and is an excellent addition to soups, stews, and other simmered dishes. This highly nutritious vegetable is perfect for juicing and blending into green smoothies, too.

TIPS AND PRECAUTIONS

Kale's taste is a little stronger than that of spinach. If you find this vegetable tastes bitter, cut the central stalks away from the kale leaves. Once you're familiar with the flavor, begin cooking some of the central stalk along with the leaves. It contains powerful nutrients that can help you stay healthy and looking your best.

If you have a history of kidney stones, eat kale fairly sparingly as it contains oxalates that contribute to the formation of these stones.

Lemons

Lemons are bright yellow citrus fruits with a zesty, fresh aroma and a tart taste. Very low in calories yet highly nutritious, lemons contain high levels of vitamin C, B vitamins, and minerals, including phosphorus. They also contain flavonoids, which are powerful antioxidants.

BENEFITS

Because lemons contain high levels of vitamin C, they are an excellent tonic for alleviating cold and flu symptoms. The vitamin C in lemons also makes them excellent for use in natural detoxification remedies. Although lemons have a sour, acidic taste, they can ease indigestion and promote gastrointestinal health. As they have an alkalizing effect on the body, lemons help to alleviate inflammation. Since they are mildly diuretic, these bright yellow fruits can also help to alleviate swelling associated with chronic conditions as well as minor injuries.

Lemon juice is an effective topical remedy for several skin conditions, including acne, eczema, and dry, cracked feet. In addition, drinking water with lemon juice promotes healthy, glowing skin. And lemon's refreshing fragrance can lift your spirits when you're feeling fatigued or mildly depressed.

HOW TO USE

Lemons are very easy to use. Simply wash them well to remove pesticide residue; then slice and use them as needed. Be sure to breathe deep when slicing into lemons, and you'll give yourself a mental boost while preparing simple remedies.

When buying lemons, look for those that are firm and glossy and avoid those with obvious soft spots or dried skin. Meyer lemons are more flavorful than other varieties, although they're often smaller; enjoy them when they are in season.

TIPS AND PRECAUTIONS

Those who suffer from frequent heartburn, gallstones, or kidney disease should use lemons sparingly and discontinue use if it causes problems to worsen.

Protect tooth enamel by waiting at least thirty minutes before brushing your teeth after ingesting a remedy that contains lemon juice.

Mushrooms

All edible mushrooms are high in minerals and vitamins, but some types contain some additional useful compounds, including polysaccharides and glycosides (carbohydrates), eritadenine (found in shiitake mushrooms, it can lower cholesterol), sterols (also help lower cholesterol), and enzymes. That means some mushrooms have more healing benefits than others.

BENEFITS

Almost all edible mushrooms are high in zinc, which is a mineral that can help lessen the duration and intensity of a common cold. When consumed regularly, they can help bolster the immune system and prevent you from getting sick as frequently as you might otherwise.

Some types of mushrooms have shown promise in helping to slow down the progress of cancer. These include reishi, shiitake, maitake, oyster mushrooms, and white button mushrooms.

HOW TO USE

Mushrooms should be wiped well with a damp paper towel before being eaten. They may be eaten raw and can be very nice in salads. However, some types, including oyster and shiitake mushrooms, are easier to digest when cooked. Mushrooms may be sautéed or baked, and they make a fantastic addition to soups, stews, and casseroles.

TIPS AND PRECAUTIONS

Select fresh mushrooms with no apparent spoiled spots, and store them in your refrigerator's crisper drawer.

Dried mushrooms are easy to reconstitute and use in recipes, and they're often less expensive per pound than fresh ones are, particularly if you want to enjoy mushrooms out of season. Canned mushrooms are available, too, but as they are highly processed, they are less desirable than fresh or dried mushrooms.

If you dislike the flavor of mushrooms but want to enjoy the health benefits that come with consuming them, you can take a mushroom supplement instead.

Though you may be tempted to forage for wild mushrooms, do so only if you are very knowledgeable in foraging and can positively identify edible mushrooms. Many deadly mushroom varieties look and smell much like edible ones, so be sure to err on the side of caution.

Nuts

Nuts are high in protein and healthful fats, plus they contain high levels of fiber, vitamins, and minerals. Easy to store and transport, nuts are a wonderfully healthful snack. They're also high in compounds that may aid in preventing serious diseases.

BENEFITS

Nuts serve as a compact energy source and can beat even serious hunger pangs in just a short amount of time. Despite the fact that they're relatively high in calories, they are ideal for anyone who is attempting to lose weight, since they help to stabilize blood sugar and cut cravings.

Nuts are also high in polyunsaturated and monounsaturated fats, which can help to reduce total cholesterol levels and keep LDL (bad) cholesterol levels in check, particularly when they are used to replace saturated fats in your daily diet.

If you suffer from dry skin, brittle nails, and dry hair that tends to break, consider eating a handful of nuts each day. Good ones to try include Brazil nuts, cashews, almonds, and walnuts.

The zinc, protein, and vitamins in nuts, especially almonds, can help improve memory while contributing to overall feelings of well-being. Different nuts also have different benefits. For example, Brazil nuts are high in selenium, which is a trace mineral that can help alleviate anxiety and depression.

HOW TO USE

Raw nuts are very good for you, but they have a tendency to spoil rather quickly. Keep them in the refrigerator. If you are looking for convenience, choose roasted nuts—preferably the low-sodium or no-salt variety. Watch portion sizes, since nuts are high in calories.

TIPS AND PRECAUTIONS

Watch out for nut products that have lots of added ingredients that might cancel out the health benefits the nuts themselves provide. For instance, many popular products contain hydrogenated or partially hydrogenated oils, which are among the worst things for your body. Some nut products contain lots of added sugar, and others have artificial flavorings added that could have a detrimental effect on your health.

If you have never eaten nuts, use caution. Nut allergies are common and can be life threatening. Try a very small amount at first to gauge whether you have any side effects. If your mouth begins to itch or your throat starts to feel tight, seek emergency treatment.

Oats

Oats are a cereal grain that has been cultivated since the Bronze Age. With a mild, nutty flavor and a pleasant, chewy consistency, these little grains are very high in both soluble and insoluble fiber, plus they contain vitamins, minerals, lipids, and a high percentage of protein.

BENEFITS

Oats are delicious, filling, and nutritious, plus they have some surprising health benefits. They contain compounds that have been found to fight cancer, reduce the risk of heart disease, improve insulin sensitivity, reduce blood sugar levels, and aid in healthful weight loss. The soluble fiber they contain helps sweep arteries clean and reduce cholesterol, and the beta-glucan they contain sweeps cholesterol from the digestive tract.

Not only are oats an excellent addition to your daily diet, but they can also be used in a variety of home remedies. If you are suffering from an itchy rash, you can prepare an oatmeal bath and relax in it; the same fiber that helps to keep your insides healthy soothes your skin and helps prevent the inflammation from becoming worse. Oatmeal baths are ideal for soothing painful rashes caused by chicken pox, poison ivy, or poison oak.

HOW TO USE

When preparing oatmeal for a meal, be sure to follow package instructions. You can also use oatmeal for an oatmeal bath.

TIPS AND PRECAUTIONS

When buying oats, be sure to select a variety that does not contain additives. Instant oatmeal products contain a wide variety of additives, from synthetic vitamins and minerals to thickeners like guar gum, artificial flavorings like malic acid, and caramel color. Stick to the basics: steel-cut (Irish) oats, rolled oats, or quick oats. Steel-cut oats are delicious, but they take longer to cook than rolled oats. Rolled oats are thicker and chewier than quick oats, and quick oats are the fastest to prepare and the best for use in oatmeal baths.

Papayas

Papayas are greenish-yellow to yellowish-orange fruits with an oblong shape, a sweet, tropical taste, and lots of black seeds. Sometimes referred to as pawpaws, papayas are rich in vitamins and minerals. They're high in fiber and low in calories, but that's just the beginning. These delicious fruits also contain the enzymes chymopapain and papain, which make papayas particularly useful for treating several common problems.

BENEFITS

Enjoy papayas a few times a week and you'll be doing your immune system a favor. People who consume this fruit regularly have been found to suffer from minor illnesses, including the flu and common colds, less often than those who do not eat it. Papayas are also excellent for preventing indigestion and bloating, particularly after large meals. The papain and chymopapain they contain help break down proteins and prevent the overgrowth of undesirable bacteria in the gastrointestinal tract.

Papayas are also known for their anti-inflammatory properties. If you suffer from osteoarthritis or rheumatoid arthritis, you may find it helpful to eat papayas regularly.

HOW TO USE

Fresh papaya should be washed well before use. To prepare it, cut it in half and scoop out the seeds. The seeds are high in protein. Though most people discard them, they can be eaten with no ill side effects. Cut the fruit into chunks and enjoy it in a fruit salad, a smoothie, or all by itself. You can also cut the papaya lengthwise and eat it right out of the skin. Many people like to dress their papaya with a squeeze of lime juice.

TIPS AND PRECAUTIONS

If fresh papaya isn't available, you may be able to find dried papaya at a supermarket near you. Look for a brand without added sugar. If you are among the few people who dislike the taste of papaya and you want to enjoy its benefits, you can take papaya supplements instead of eating the fruit.

Peppermint

Peppermint is an aromatic plant with a cool, refreshing flavor. It gets its delightful fragrance and its pleasant taste from the high percentage of menthol it contains.

BENEFITS

Peppermint is such a beneficial food that it treats almost everything. It is excellent for alleviating nausea and indigestion, and it is a wonderful remedy for relieving annoying cold symptoms such as a cough and sore throat.

The uplifting fragrance of peppermint soothes the spirit and can brighten even the sourest mood. It can also help to promote alertness and enhance memory.

When applied to the skin, the herb relieves itching associated with hives and rashes. A compress made from peppermint leaves is an effective remedy for tension and sinus headaches.

Peppermint is also an excellent natural breath freshener, and when enjoyed after a meal, it can help alleviate cravings for sweets.

HOW TO USE

The easiest way to use peppermint is as tea. To make it, simply steep fresh or dried peppermint leaves in boiling water until the water has cooled enough to be sipped. Peppermint can also be made into a compress. To freshen breath naturally, simply chew on fresh peppermint leaves or enjoy a refreshing cup of peppermint tea.

TIPS AND PRECAUTIONS

If you suffer from a hiatal hernia or from gastroesophageal reflux disease (GERD), peppermint can make your symptoms worse and should not be used. If you have an unusual stomach condition called achlorhydria, peppermint oil in pill form may dissolve too early in the digestive process to be useful.

Pineapple

Spiny but sweet, pineapple is a delicious tropical fruit that's often considered a treat rather than a nutritional powerhouse. Pineapple is an outstanding source of vitamins and minerals, along with antioxidants and enzymes.

BENEFITS

Besides promoting general well-being, pineapple is an excellent food for reducing inflammation and promoting healing. If you've had surgery, are on the mend with a broken bone, or are recuperating from a sprain or minor illness, the bromelain (enzyme) in pineapple can help to expedite your recovery. The fruit is an excellent choice for promoting healthy joints, healthy blood vessels, and a healthy heart.

The enzymes in pineapple help facilitate healthy digestion, and they break down proteins quickly. They can also aid in reducing gas and bloating, and can ease constipation.

Why It Works Bromelain digests protein, making it a welcome digestive aid when you've overeaten. This property also makes it effective in removing dead skin from a wound or burn, and in reducing swelling after physical injuries. Bromelain is a particularly effective healing agent for surgery involving the sinuses.

HOW TO USE

While processed pineapple and pineapple juice often cost less than fresh pineapple, you'll obtain more health benefits from ripe, fresh pineapple than you will from canned or bottled products. Eat pineapple any time, or add it to smoothies. It's also ideal for making your own fresh juice.

If preparing fresh pineapple seems like a hassle, you can buy it peeled and cut—but still fresh—in many grocery stores. Pineapple bromelain supplements are available at health food stores and online.

While fresh pineapple is delicious and healthful, some people are allergic or sensitive to it. If you eat excessive amounts of pineapple, you may feel a tingling sensation in your mouth and also suffer from diarrhea.

Pineapple and pineapple juice can increase the effects of prescription blood thinners. If you are on blood-thinning medication and want to enjoy pineapple or take pineapple supplements, be sure to talk with your doctor first to make sure it is safe.

Red Wine

Like many of the foods we love, red wine also has the power to heal the body and improve overall health. Red wine is made from dark grape varieties and contains high levels of antioxidants, including resveratrol, which is believed to protect the lining of blood vessels in the heart while reducing "bad" LDL cholesterol. Red wine is also a good source of naturally occurring fluoride.

BENEFITS

The antioxidants in red wine aid in preventing heart disease by reducing the risk of arterial damage and increasing HDL (good) cholesterol levels. The resveratrol it contains helps reduce the risk of developing blood clots and aids in preventing heart attack and stroke.

Resveratrol also helps protect the body from carcinogens and can slow the spread of cancer cell growth. It can also slow the growth of existing tumors while helping to prevent existing cancer cells from mutating and becoming resistant to chemotherapy.

Red wine is also an excellent medium for making herbal decoctions, as the alcohol it contains aids in extracting healing compounds from plant structures.

HOW TO USE

While many healing foods should be eaten in large quantities, red wine should be enjoyed in moderation, as it is high in sugar and calories—and alcohol. Drinking too much wine can negate the health benefits it offers. The American Heart Association recommends that people consume no more than one to two glasses of red wine a day to gain the greatest benefits—one glass for women, and two for men. It's important to drink your wine over time—consuming a few days' worth at one time will not benefit you and may do more harm than good.

Begin by choosing a red wine variety that you enjoy. Today's winemakers have perfected their craft, and even less expensive wines are often very good. Open the wine and pour it into glasses, ensuring that you stick to a moderate four- to five-ounce serving size. Allow the glasses of wine to sit for about five minutes so the wine has a chance to "breathe" (that is, oxidize) and develop optimal flavor before you start sipping.

Wine is best enjoyed as an accompaniment to food. Different wines pair well with different types of food. When shopping for wines, ask at your local shop or research online in advance, so you know what wines to choose to complement your dinner menu.

TIPS AND PRECAUTIONS

If you are susceptible to migraines, you might not be able to drink red wine, as it can be a trigger. Different wines act differently in various individuals, though, and not all migraine sufferers are susceptible to headaches caused by red wine.

When you drink, be sure to do so responsibly. Choose a designated driver or stay home to enjoy your wine. If friends are drinking with you, be sure they are sober before allowing them to drive home.

Yogurt

Yogurt, whether dairy or nondairy, Greek or French, is creamy and tangy. It is high in protein, rich in calcium, and perfect for blending with everything from savory herbs to sweet fruit or honey. It also happens to be one of the few foods that contain probiotics—organisms that help maintain the natural balance of microflora in the intestines. Other essential nutrients include B vitamins, vitamin D, magnesium, and potassium.

BENEFITS

Yogurt with live, active cultures benefits digestion and can help restore balance to the gastrointestinal tract after a bout with diarrhea or food poisoning. The probiotics in yogurt can also help keep the body's immunity levels high.

During or after a course of antibiotics, yogurt can help replenish the intestinal microflora destroyed by the antibiotics.

If you're suffering from diarrhea or constipation, eating yogurt can help restore balance and bring bowel movements back to normal. If you have stomach ulcers, yogurt may help relieve the discomfort and help keep excess acid in check.

Women who tend to suffer from frequent yeast infections can reduce the number and severity of infections by eating yogurt with no added sugar regularly. If a yeast infection is active, plain yogurt may even be applied topically. If the infection worsens or does not clear up within three days, visit your doctor.

Yogurt can soothe sunburns, smooth and moisturize skin, and fight dandruff, and is an excellent addition to homemade facial masks and scrubs.

HOW TO USE

Yogurt may be eaten plain or with fruit and honey. It can also be strained through cheesecloth to make a delicious low-fat cheese, and it's perfect for use in many of your favorite recipes. Dairy and nondairy yogurt are wonderful additions to fruit smoothies, and plain varieties can be used to replace fatty sour cream.

When applying yogurt topically, scoop the desired amount out into a small dish and use a cotton ball or cotton pad to apply it to the area you are treating. Be sure to wipe up any spills immediately, as spoiled yogurt has an undesirable odor.

TIPS AND PRECAUTIONS

When buying yogurt for home remedies, be sure to choose a brand that contains live, active cultures, including *Streptococcus thermophilus* and *Lactobacillus bulgaricus*. Yogurt that is used topically should be plain, with no added fruit, sugar, or artificial sweeteners.

Either Greek yogurt or regular yogurt will work for the remedies found in this book, and remedies you'll find elsewhere, unless otherwise specified. If you're buying yogurt for consumption, you'll find that nonfat Greek yogurt is more nutritious, with double the protein of regular yogurt and a richer, creamier taste that many people find irresistible.

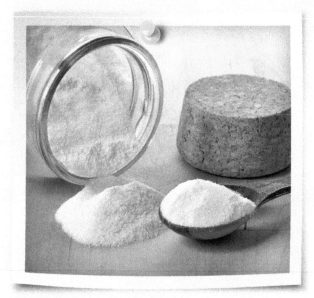

HEALING HOUSEHOLD PRODUCTS

- Aloe Vera Gel
- Apple Cider Vinegar
- Aspirin
- Baking Soda
- Borax
- Coffee
- Cornstarch

- Epsom Salt
- Hydrogen Peroxide
- Ice
- Menthol Rub
- Mineral Oil
- Mouthwash
- Olive Oil
- Oral Anesthetic Gel

- Pink Bismuth
- Rubbing Alcohol
- Salt
- Toothpaste
- Witch Hazel

CHAPTER 4

Healing Household Products

Many common household products can be used to make effective home remedies for everything from acne to warts. Often extremely inexpensive, these items can be found in your kitchen cupboard, your bathroom medicine cabinet, and even your desk. Although some of the remedies found here may seem a little unusual to you, they have been tested and will work well most of the time.

You'll notice that many of the household products mentioned in this chapter have a variety of uses. For example, apple cider vinegar can be used to soothe sunburns, remove stains from teeth, make your hair shinier, and more. Not only does this help you maximize cupboard space and clear clutter, it also helps you save money by reducing the need for countless products and potions intended for just a single purpose.

While home remedies made with household products can often be effective, sometimes they fail to produce the desired action. If your condition worsens despite treatment at home, be sure to seek medical help to prevent it from becoming a major problem.

Aloe Vera Gel

Aloe vera gel is found inside the leaves of the aloe vera plant—a succulent. Slightly sticky, with a thick, jelly-like texture, the gel has a cooling effect.

BENEFITS

Aloe vera gel can be used to treat minor burns, cuts, and scrapes. In addition, it can reduce the appearance of scars, including acne scars. When used regularly, it can also help reduce the appearance of wrinkles.

Aloe gel is an effective treatment for scalp itch, and it can also help to alleviate itching and irritation caused by insect bites, bee stings, and contact with poisonous plants, including poison ivy.

Why It Works Aloe gel contains polysaccharides, which speed skin growth and repair, and glycoproteins, which assist in the healing process by alleviating pain, irritation, and inflammation. These combined attributes make aloe gel a powerful ally in wound recovery.

HOW TO USE

You can buy aloe vera gel at drugstores and health food stores, and it can also be obtained from living aloe plants that are four years old or older. Though younger plants produce the gel, they do not recover from the trauma of removing leaves as well as older plants do.

To treat minor burns and other minor skin injuries, including stings, bites, rashes, and minor sunburn, simply wash the affected area thoroughly with cool water and apply the aloe vera gel. Cover with a bandage, if needed.

TIPS AND PRECAUTIONS

When obtaining aloe vera gel from a living plant, be sure to harvest the oldest, outermost leaves, since they contain the most gel and new leaves come from the central portion of the plant. Use just what you need and store the rest in the refrigerator for up to a week, using it for subsequent treatments.

Although aloe gel may be taken internally, it has a strong laxative effect and is not recommended for long-term use.

Apple Cider Vinegar

Apple cider vinegar is made from apple juice that has been fermented to make hard cider. The hard cider is fermented a second time to make the vinegar, which is highly acidic, and which contains high levels of antioxidants and pectin.

BENEFITS

Apple cider vinegar is traditionally used for making pickles and other foods, but when used as a remedy, it does more than brighten flavors. Not only does it aid in keeping blood glucose levels stable, it also helps prevent high blood pressure.

HOW TO USE

You can use apple cider vinegar in a bath to treat sunburn. Aid detoxification by sipping a liter of water that has two tablespoons of apple cider vinegar added to it. Keep sipping all day to help remove toxins from the body. As an added benefit, this apple cider vinegar remedy is an effective aid to natural weight loss, particularly when paired with a healthful, balanced diet and regular exercise.

TIPS AND PRECAUTIONS

WebMD found a range of additives in the brands of apple cider vinegar they analyzed. They also found that some brands may not even contain apple cider. Read the bottle label carefully to be sure you're buying the purest possible vinegar.

Dilute pure apple cider vinegar with water when it's taken orally, as it is highly acidic and can damage tooth enamel and tissues in your throat and mouth. In some cases it has also been known to burn the skin. Consuming eight ounces of apple cider vinegar per day over the long term can reduce potassium levels in your body, which can lead to high blood pressure. This kind of use also may weaken your bones—a sign of osteoporosis—and lower your blood sugar levels. Consult your doctor before using apple cider vinegar if you have osteoporosis, diabetes, or low potassium levels.

Aspirin

Aspirin is an effective analgesic with astringent and anti-inflammatory properties. It inhibits blood clotting and is antipyretic, meaning it is capable of reducing fever.

BENEFITS

Not only is aspirin effective for pain relief when taken orally, it can also be used for several other purposes. Reduce the appearance of pimples and make them less painful, soften calluses, and soothe insect bites and bee stings with aspirin.

HOW TO USE

Make a paste by crushing adult aspirin tablets and mixing them with water to treat acne, soothe insect bites and bee stings, and soften calluses.

TIPS AND PRECAUTIONS

Be sure to use adult aspirin tablets for these remedies, as baby aspirin or children's aspirin has added sugar and flavorings that can adversely affect the outcome. In addition, be sure to buy plain, uncoated aspirin for use in home remedies; the coated type will not work as well, as it is difficult to crush.

Do not give aspirin to children for any reason, unless you are advised to do so by a medical professional. Aspirin use in children has been linked closely to Reye's syndrome, a rare illness that children can develop while they are recovering from the flu, a cold, or chicken pox. The syndrome causes the brain to swell and can lead to liver failure, brain damage, or death. Between 1979 and 1980, the peak of Reye's syndrome's emergence, 90 to 95 percent of the cases involved children who had been given aspirin while they had the flu or a cold. Cases are very scarce now that parents no longer give their children aspirin during these illnesses.

Some people have an allergy or sensitivity to aspirin. This may also apply to topical preparations. If you have a problem with aspirin, try just a tiny amount of paste on your skin. Wash it off immediately with plenty of water if you notice any reaction.

Baking Soda

Also known as sodium bicarbonate, baking soda is an alkaline substance, meaning it balances acids. It was originally derived from natural natron, which ancient Egyptians used as a cleansing and embalming agent. Today's baking soda is produced using a simple chemical process that relies on the reaction of ammonia, sodium chloride, and carbon dioxide with water. Not only is the resulting product useful for baking, it is also used for everything from absorbing odors to extinguishing small fires.

BENEFITS

Because baking soda has alkalizing properties, it is very useful for neutralizing acid, which is why it has long been prized as a home remedy for soothing indigestion and relieving insect bites. As it is mildly abrasive, it is useful for keeping teeth bright and white. Its ability to absorb scents makes it ideal for reducing foot odors and other noxious smells.

HOW TO USE

Baking soda can be dissolved in water, made into a thick paste, or applied directly in its powdered form, depending on the remedy.

TIPS AND PRECAUTIONS

Baking soda can decrease the body's absorption of certain medications, including the antibiotic tetracycline. If you take prescription medications, be sure to talk with your doctor before ingesting baking soda (although topical preparations are fine). In addition, do not take baking soda orally within two hours of taking vitamins or over-the-counter medications by mouth, as baking soda can reduce the efficacy of the vitamins or medication.

Be sure to buy a fresh box of baking soda to use for home remedies rather than using an old box that has been in your refrigerator or cupboard for some time. Keep baking soda fresh by storing it in a sealed container. This will prevent lumps from forming, and it will prevent the baking soda from absorbing odors from other items stored nearby.

Borax

Also known as sodium borate, borax is a common ingredient in soaps, including laundry detergent. This white, colorless salt dissolves easily in water and has antifungal, antiviral, and disinfecting properties.

BENEFITS

You might know that borax is useful for whitening laundry and keeping your house clean naturally, but that's not all it's good for. You can also use borax to stop foot fungus and eliminate athlete's foot.

HOW TO USE

A borax foot soak will help treat your athlete's foot. You can add a few drops of your favorite essential oil to the footbath for a pleasant scent—some favorites include lavender, peppermint, and eucalyptus.

TIPS AND PRECAUTIONS

Do not confuse borax with boric acid. Borax occurs naturally, while boric acid is a chemical compound made from borax. You'll find powdered borax for sale at drugstores and big-box stores, usually in the laundry aisle. The mineral can also be used for killing fleas in carpets, as long as you don't have cats—your cats have a natural sensitivity to borax and will develop breathing problems. In some cases, borax can be fatal to cats.

Coffee

Not only is coffee a favorite morning beverage with the power to wake people up, it is also an effective remedy for a number of minor problems. Coffee contains caffeine, which is a type of alkaloid that acts as a stimulant.

BENEFITS

Coffee is such an effective stimulant that people all over the world rely on it for help waking up in the morning and for preventing late-day sleepiness. But coffee is also a useful ingredient in a number of effective home remedies. For example, it can remove odors such as garlic, onion, or fish from the hands. Just rub a little ground coffee between your palms for about twenty seconds and rinse—strong odors will disappear.

The caffeine in coffee acts as a vasodilator, making it a good remedy for firming the skin and reducing the appearance of cellulite. Finely ground coffee beans are useful as an exfoliant that leaves skin glowing. You can also use coffee as a nourishing rinse for your hair.

Why It Works Caffeine not only is a stimulant but also contains nitrogen, a key ingredient that cleans unpleasant smells from the air. Brewed coffee grounds, with their concentration of caffeine and nitrogen, will clean odors from your hands, out of your kitchen, and away from your trash.

HOW TO USE

When preparing coffee as a beverage, simply brew it according to the instructions that came with your coffeemaker. Coffee grounds can also be used as a scrub for the skin or a poultice for reducing the appearance of cellulite. Brewed espresso makes an excellent rinse for shinier, softer hair.

TIPS AND PRECAUTIONS

People with heart disease and high blood pressure should limit their consumption of caffeine, and some may not be able to drink it at all. Do not use coffee remedies if your doctor has directed you to avoid caffeine.

Caffeine is a natural stimulant, and can interfere with sleep patterns. If you find this is the case for you, stick to topical preparations after the morning.

Cornstarch

Cornstarch is derived from the endosperm of corn kernels, and is typically used to thicken soups and sauces. When used in home remedies, it is great for absorbing toxins, oils, and excess moisture as well as for calming itchy skin.

BENEFITS

Cornstarch is an excellent cosmetic remedy that can be useful for absorbing excess oil. It can be used to keep oily skin from looking overly shiny, and it can be used as a dry shampoo that absorbs excess oil from the scalp when you don't have time to wash and condition your hair.

Because of its ability to relieve itching, cornstarch is an excellent remedy for hives and insect bites. You can either soak in a bath containing cornstarch, or you can make a simple paste from it and apply it to the affected areas.

Cornstarch can also be used to treat diaper rash. Since it soothes skin and absorbs moisture, it is ideal for use on tender skin.

HOW TO USE

In most cases, cornstarch can be used dry and simply patted or shaken onto the affected area. Use it to remove excess oil from the skin and hair. Treat a baby's diaper rash and keep the affected area dry by sprinkling on cornstarch, When using it to absorb excess oil from skin, you can either apply it with a cosmetic sponge or a brush. Make a paste of cornstarch and water for insect bites, hives, and other itches.

The moisture-absorbing properties also make cornstarch good for staunching the bleeding from minor cuts and scrapes. Place a little bit directly on the cut and the bleeding will stop.

TIPS AND PRECAUTIONS

Store your cornstarch in a sealed container in a cool, dry place. This will prevent lumps from forming.

When exposed to water, cornstarch can form a lumpy paste and blend unevenly. Solve this problem by adding cool or room temperature water to the starch gradually, whisking it thoroughly as you go; avoid hot water, because it will cause the cornstarch to coagulate.

Do not apply dry shampoo made with cornstarch to damp or wet hair. This will cause a mess that you'll need to shampoo out. Be sure all dry shampoo has been removed from your hair before adding other styling products, such as mousse or hairspray, since these products can also cause the starch to clump.

Epsom Salt

Also known as bitter salt or magnesium sulfate, Epsom salt is a chemical compound that contains magnesium, oxygen, and sulfur. Though its crystals look much like table salt, Epsom salt is usually used externally. It is primarily useful for its anti-inflammatory and detoxification properties.

BENEFITS

Epsom salt reduces inflammation, softens skin, and can soothe sore, tired muscles. It also aids in detoxification, stress relief, and pain relief. When taken internally, Epsom salt can be used as a laxative.

HOW TO USE

Epsom salt can be mixed with water and drunk as a laxative. To ease pain and promote detoxification, simply enjoy a warm bath with a half-cup of Epsom salt added. Remain in the bathtub for fifteen to thirty minutes, relaxing and breathing deeply. Add two or three drops of your favorite essential oil to the bath to enhance the experience.

For soaking the feet to reduce swelling, add one cup of Epsom salt to one gallon of warm water. Soak your feet (or hands) for fifteen to twenty minutes.

TIPS AND PRECAUTIONS

People who are allergic to sulfur should avoid contact with Epsom salt. Epsom salt baths can also be harmful to those who have high blood pressure or suffer from cardiovascular disease. People who have diabetes, adrenal issues, and thyroid problems should consult their physician before using Epsom salt.

Use of Epsom salt topically—as an additive to bath water or as a foot soak, for example—is considered safe for pregnant women. This usage can reduce the swelling in ankles and feet that so many pregnant women experience. Avoid using Epsom salt as a laxative while you are pregnant, however, as the salt works by shifting fluids from other parts of your body into your intestines. This process can cause cramping and even start premature contractions.

Hydrogen Peroxide

Hydrogen peroxide is a clear liquid that is used as a cleanser and disinfectant. It is strongly reactive, with oxidizing properties that make it mildly corrosive. While pure hydrogen peroxide is unstable and is not commercially available, mild hydrogen peroxide solutions are available at drugstores and are suitable for use in a number of home remedies.

BENEFITS

Hydrogen peroxide is a powerful germicidal agent and sanitizer. When it reacts with organic material, it simply breaks down into its original components, which are water and oxygen. Hydrogen peroxide can be used to soften feet and eliminate foot fungus. It can also be used in a detoxifying bath that softens skin, and it is an effective treatment for canker sores, sore gums, and halitosis.

HOW TO USE

Hydrogen peroxide can be used topically to clean minor wounds. Rinse the wound well with water, then rinse it with hydrogen peroxide. Allow the peroxide to work for about thirty seconds, then rinse the wound with water again before applying antibiotic ointment and a bandage. This treatment can help slow bleeding and lift small particles of debris from wounds. Mix the hydrogen peroxide with water and spray it on to fight foot fungus. A peroxide-and-water soak helps soften skin. And a little swish can tame bad breath.

TIPS AND PRECAUTIONS

While hydrogen peroxide can be used to clean wounds, it should not be left in contact with broken skin for longer than about thirty seconds, since it can damage living tissue and slow the healing process. If you have a serious wound or a wound that is filled with debris, hydrogen peroxide is most likely not going to be enough to treat it. While it may help with first aid, it is not a suitable replacement for proper medical treatment.

You can swish with hydrogen peroxide to help eliminate halitosis, but be careful not to swallow it. A small amount won't hurt you, but more than about half a teaspoon can cause complications with digestion.

Ice

Ice is simply frozen water. As it has strong cooling capabilities, it can ease inflammation, eliminate itching, and reduce swelling.

BENEFITS

Simple ice offers many wonderful benefits. It can help reduce fever, aid in cooling the body, and increase circulation to promote healing. It is an excellent remedy for soothing pain, reducing swelling, and reducing the redness and pain associated with bruises. Ice can also help ease pain and itching associated with insect bites and bee stings.

HOW TO USE

When you're suffering from a fever or are very hot, drink a beverage with ice to help bring your body temperature down. Treat minor burns, minor sprains, and bruises with ice packs applied directly to the injury site. Elevate the area if possible to help promote circulation, and leave the ice packs in place for fifteen to thirty minutes at a time, repeating as needed to help promote healing.

You can use ice packs on bug bites and bee stings, as well. Apply the ice pack as soon after the sting as possible to increase circulation and promote detoxification. The cooling effect of the ice acts as a mild anesthetic, helping to ease the pain and itch that accompany stings and bites.

If someone is seriously overheated or suffering a fever higher than 103 degrees Fahrenheit or any fever that doesn't break, seek medical treatment, particularly if the victim seems to be disoriented or if he or she is convulsing or unconscious. When using an ice pack to treat wounds and insect stings, wrap it in a soft cloth to protect the skin from freezing. If a body part cannot bear weight or any pressure, seek medical attention. While ice can be used to soothe minor burns, seek medical treatment for large burns and burns with blistering or broken skin.

Menthol Rub

Sometimes referred to as chest rub or vapor rub, menthol rub is a petroleum-based gel that contains menthol. Though originally intended to soothe coughs and colds, menthol rub has mild anesthetic properties that make it ideal for treating skin irritations.

BENEFITS

Menthol rub alleviates the stinging and itching associated with insect bites and bee stings. It can also be used as a topical analgesic for soothing sore joints and muscles, and as it has a cooling effect, it is sometimes effective for alleviating the discomfort associated with hemorrhoids.

Because menthol rub contains petroleum jelly, it can help to soothe cracked, dry skin, including cracked heels.

HOW TO USE

To treat insect bites, bee stings, sore muscles and joints, and dry skin, simply apply a small amount of menthol rub to the affected area. When treating dry, cracked skin on feet, be sure to wear socks so you don't slip and fall, and so the menthol rub remains in contact with your skin.

Reapply the menthol rub as needed for all treatments, watching for potential irritation that menthol sometimes causes.

Although there's an old wives tale that recommends ingesting menthol rub mixed with warm milk, this treatment is ineffective and can be dangerous. Menthol rub is intended for topical use only.

Mineral Oil

Also known as baby oil, mineral oil is a lightweight, transparent oil that has long been used to help keep skin soft. It is noncomedogenic, meaning it does not block the skin's pores, making it a popular ingredient in cosmetics.

BENEFITS

Mineral oil can be used to help hold moisture in, and it can also act as a barrier between the elements and the skin, making it a good choice for application during cold, dry winter weather. It fights dishpan hands and can even help prevent stretch marks.

It is also useful for clearing excess wax from the ears, removing sticky bandages, and removing gum from kids' hair. You can also use it to remove makeup, including eye makeup.

Why It Works Mineral oil is a byproduct of the process of turning petroleum into gasoline. The oil is a close cousin of petroleum jelly, with the added advantage of being a liquid—perfect for lubricating metals and woods . . . and removing chewing gum in hair.

HOW TO USE

Mineral oil can be used as a moisturizer in a few different ways. You can add a tablespoon or so to a warm bath, apply it to your skin after showering, or slather it on exposed skin before heading out into freezing cold weather. You can apply it to your hands after doing dishes, while the skin is still damp, and your hands will remain soft and supple instead of developing scaly, dry patches.

To clear excess wax from your ears, drip two or three drops of mineral oil into your ears, one at a time. Lie on your side for a few minutes, allowing the mineral oil to remain in your ear. Switch sides to allow the mineral oil and accumulated wax to drain out, placing a towel under your head to catch the oil and debris that come out.

If you have a bandage that's stuck on tight, you can use mineral oil to remove it painlessly. Just soak a cotton ball in mineral oil and rub around the edges of the bandage. Keep rubbing at the adhesive as the bandage loosens, and within a few moments, you'll be bandage-free.

You can also use mineral oil to remove gum that's stuck in hair. Gently apply mineral oil to the affected area and allow it to sit for about a minute. The gum should come right out. Use additional mineral oil to work out any remaining bits of gum; then wash, condition, and dry your hair as usual.

TIPS AND PRECAUTIONS

Mineral oil is extremely slippery. If you use it when bathing or showering, be careful, as it can accumulate on bath and shower floors. Wipe up any drips and excess with a towel to prevent falls.

If you buy unscented mineral oil, you can make your own scented bath and body oil by using your favorite essential oil. Just mix in a drop or two, making sure the essential oil you choose is safe to apply to skin. Some nice combinations are peppermint and eucalyptus, lavender and vanilla, and lavender and peppermint.

Mouthwash

Mouthwash freshens breath, and because of its high alcohol content, it acts as an effective germicide and fungicide. It also has anti-inflammatory properties.

BENEFITS

Not only does mouthwash help put a stop to halitosis, it can also be used to treat minor cuts and scrapes, and it can be used to kill foot fungus and halt athlete's foot. Mouthwash can also help minimize the appearance of bruises, and since it helps to ease inflammation, it can be used to take the sting out of insect bites, hives, and rashes.

HOW TO USE

If you have a minor cut or scrape, you can disinfect it by applying mouthwash with a cotton swab or cotton ball, or by pouring a small amount of mouthwash over the affected area. Brace yourself, because the alcohol is going to cause the area to sting for a moment after the mouthwash has been applied. The trade-off is a clean wound that is less likely to become infected. Either allow the area to dry and form a scab, or treat it with antibiotic ointment and cover it with a bandage.

When you're in need of an emergency treatment for a bee sting, itchy mosquito bites, hives, or a rash—including one caused by contact with poison ivy—mouthwash can help alleviate the itch. Use a cotton swab or cotton balls to apply the mouthwash to the affected area. If the rash covers a large area, apply the mouthwash with a soft cloth.

TIPS AND PRECAUTIONS

Choose sugar-free mouthwash made with alcohol for these remedies, since the alcohol is what makes the treatments effective.

Olive Oil

Olive oil has long been used in cosmetics, soaps, and pharmaceuticals. It is a wonderful moisturizer with soothing and protective properties.

BENEFITS

Olive oil is great for cooking, and it's also excellent for treating dry skin and softening hair, soothing chapped lips, and easing diaper rash. Olive oil can also be used for oil pulling, which is a natural detoxification remedy that can also help prevent gingivitis and tooth decay.

HOW TO USE

Have about a tablespoon of olive oil each day, either in a soup, on a salad, or as a healthful dip for your bread, and you'll be nourishing your body from the inside out. Olive oil is among the most healthful fats you can consume, and eating it regularly contributes to healthful HDL (good) cholesterol levels, healthy arteries, and soft, supple skin.

You can apply a few drops of olive oil to chapped lips to soften them and aid healing, and you can use olive oil to moisturize skin, too. Pay careful attention to very dry patches of skin, including those on the knees and elbows, applying a little extra olive oil to those areas.

For oil pulling—an ancient Ayurveda treatment for oral health and detoxification—place one tablespoon of cold-pressed olive oil in your mouth first thing in the morning before eating or drinking anything. Do not swallow the oil. Instead, slowly pull it through your mouth, pulling it between all of your teeth and allowing it to mix with saliva as you go. The first time you do this, you may be able to do it for only a minute or two. Gradually increase the amount of time you spend on this process, working your way up to twenty minutes each morning. Spit the oil out when you are finished, then rinse your mouth with water and go about your day. Sunflower oil, sesame oil, and coconut oil are also good choices for oil pulling.

TIPS AND PRECAUTIONS

Read olive oil labels carefully when shopping, and make sure you select a brand that contains no additives or preservatives. Since light can damage olive oil, choose a brand that comes packaged in a dark container.

Oral Anesthetic Gel

This over-the-counter oral anesthetic is sold under several brand names and store names, including Anbesol and Orajel. It contains benzocaine, which is a topical numbing agent.

BENEFITS

Not only is oral anesthetic gel useful for inhibiting minor dental pain, it can also be used to soothe itching caused by insect bites, ease the burn of a bee sting, and alleviate discomfort caused by minor burns.

HOW TO USE

If you have suffered a minor burn, have itchy mosquito bites, or have a bee sting, simply dab some oral anesthetic gel onto the affected area and leave it there. Reapply as needed.

TIPS AND PRECAUTIONS

Some people are sensitive to benzocaine. If you notice redness or swelling, wash the oral anesthetic gel off your skin, being careful to remove it all.

Pink Bismuth

Pink bismuth is an effective anti-inflammatory and skin brightener, though it may be best known for its calming antacid effect—and for its color. Because it is bactericidal and an effective antacid, pink bismuth has been primarily used for eliminating diarrhea, soothing an upset stomach, and easing heartburn.

BENEFITS

Pink bismuth is helpful for shrinking pimples and brightening dull skin. It is also a good remedy for alleviating occasional indigestion. You can even use it on a bee sting if you don't have another remedy available.

Why It Works Salicylic acid is an active ingredient in pink bismuth and used in many topical acne preparations. Bismuth subsalicylate produces an oligodynamic effect–small doses have a toxic effect on microbes. Specifically, salicylic acid is the antimicrobial that works on *E. coli,* a pathogen that causes diarrhea in travelers.

HOW TO USE

To use pink bismuth as a topical anti-inflammatory, dab the liquid form on your face with a cotton ball to brighten your complexion, and on affected areas of the skin to ease the itch and sting of an insect encounter. When using pink bismuth for diarrhea or as an antacid, always follow the dosages specified on the pink bismuth bottle. Note that multiple doses are usually required for these conditions, often within an hour or less of each other. For best results, take the doses as recommended by the manufacturer.

TIPS AND PRECAUTIONS

Some people are extremely sensitive to salicylic acid. If you feel a burning sensation or begin to notice pain or swelling, rinse the pink bismuth from your skin immediately, as you could be having an adverse reaction.

Rubbing Alcohol

Rubbing alcohol is antiviral and antibacterial, and is an excellent disinfectant. Often it costs less than a dollar a bottle; this is one affordable remedy you should not be without.

BENEFITS

Anyone who has ever had to endure a finger stick or needle prick knows that rubbing alcohol is used to disinfect the site before the needle goes in. In addition, this pungent liquid can be used to disinfect hands, treat cold sores, and make flexible homemade ice packs for treating sprains and other minor injuries.

HOW TO USE

To disinfect hands, wash them with soap and water, dry them, and then splash them with a small amount of rubbing alcohol. Rub them vigorously back and forth until the alcohol dries. Apply a dab of your favorite hand lotion afterward to prevent excessively dry skin.

Homemade ice packs are very easy to make and can be used for keeping lunches cold as well as for treating minor injuries. Buy sturdy freezer bags that seal tightly and fill them with one part rubbing alcohol to three parts fresh water, leaving about an inch of empty space inside for the liquid to expand when it freezes. Freeze on a cookie sheet overnight to ensure they remain flat; then store the ice packs in the freezer.

TIPS AND PRECAUTIONS

Rubbing alcohol is not consumable. It is also not suitable for making tinctures, unless those remedies are meant for topical application only. If you accidentally ingest rubbing alcohol, seek medical treatment *immediately,* as ingestion can cause organ failure and death.

Salt

Common table salt is a crystalline mineral compound that is essential for all animal life, including humans. It is a necessary nutrient, a tasty food seasoning, and an effective antibacterial agent—which is why it has been used as a food preservative for centuries.

BENEFITS

Salt's antibacterial properties make it perfect for treating minor infections, including sore throats. As it is a drying agent, it is also useful for treating puffiness, including puffy bags that tend to pop up under tired eyes.

HOW TO USE

For home remedies like those for sore throat and puffy eyes, salt is typically mixed with water. As the salt water bathes the affected area, it draws out swelling and inflammation.

TIPS AND PRECAUTIONS

Although salt is an antibacterial agent that can help kill germs, it shouldn't be used to treat wounds, as it can cause extreme pain (hence the expression, "that hurts like rubbing salt into the wound"). In an emergency situation where salt is the only cleansing agent you have on hand, you can create a sterile saline solution by combining ¼ teaspoon of salt with one cup of water, boiling the mixture, and then allowing it to cool before use.

Toothpaste

Toothpaste is an effective cleanser with strong astringent properties. Many types of toothpaste are mildly abrasive, and most contain fluoride. Some brands of toothpaste also contain surfactants, which improve their cleansing power, and several brands have an antibacterial agent called zinc chloride or triclosan. Most also contain flavoring, with mint among the most popular.

BENEFITS

Toothpaste doesn't just help prevent cavities while keeping teeth sparkling clean; it is also an effective remedy for eliminating blackheads and whiteheads. You can also use toothpaste to alleviate itching caused by mosquito and chigger bites.

HOW TO USE

Typically, you just dab toothpaste on the affected area of the skin, leave it there for up to twenty-five minutes, and rinse it off with warm water. It doesn't get much easier!

Dermatologists have found that it is the whitening agents in toothpaste, like hydrogen peroxide and baking soda, that dry out pimples, as do the menthol and triclosan—an antibacterial—which are found in most toothpastes.

Choose white, non-gel toothpaste for topical remedies. Be careful to try the paste on a spot that isn't very visible first, as your skin may be sensitive to the ingredients in your toothpaste, and you may develop redness and peeling. A study published in the *Journal of Clinical and Aesthetic Dermatology* discovered that most allergic reactions were caused by the flavorings in the toothpaste—especially the mint varieties. This may make finding the right toothpaste for acne a little tricky.

Witch Hazel

Witch hazel is derived from the leaves, bark, and twigs of the witch hazel plant, and is an effective astringent that contains high levels of tannins, along with flavonoids that make it excellent for use as an anti-inflammatory agent.

BENEFITS

Witch hazel refreshes the skin while tightening pores and removing excess oil. It is also excellent for shrinking swollen tissues, which makes it an effective remedy for soothing discomfort caused by varicose veins and hemorrhoids. It is suitable for treating sore, swollen gums, and it can even help soothe the pain associated with laryngitis and sore throats.

Why It Works Astringents constrict or shrink body tissues, so the tannins in witch hazel can pull excretions (like oils) away from the skin to tighten the skin and calm savage acne. This ability to constrict tissues makes witch hazel an excellent choice for reducing swelling, as well.

HOW TO USE

Witch hazel is usually applied topically by simply dabbing it on with a cotton ball. But if you want to use it for swollen gums or for alleviating pain from a sore throat or laryngitis, it can be used as a mouth rinse or gargle. If you're using witch hazel tincture, dilute a medicine dropper full in ¼ cup of cool water and swish or gargle for thirty seconds. If you're using distilled liquid witch hazel (the type normally found at drugstores, which does not come with a dropper), use ½ teaspoon per ¼ cup of water.

When using witch hazel as a skin toner or as a tonic for treating varicose veins or hemorrhoids, it is best to leave it undiluted. Simply cleanse the affected area with soap and water and rinse before applying the witch hazel with a cotton pad. There is no need to rinse afterward.

TIPS AND PRECAUTIONS

A little witch hazel goes a long way. It's better to apply a small amount and need to apply a bit more than it is to apply too much and find yourself dabbing off the excess.

When applying witch hazel to your face, be careful not to get it in your eyes, as it can cause irritation.

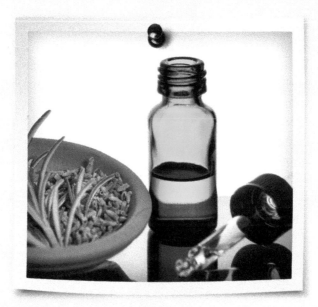

HEALING ESSENTIAL OILS

- Basil Essential Oil
- Chamomile Essential Oil
- Clary Sage Essential Oil
- Eucalyptus Essential Oil
- Frankincense Essential Oil
- Geranium Essential Oil
- Ginger Essential Oil
- Grapefruit Essential Oil
- Helichrysum Essential Oil
- Lavender Essential Oil
- Lemon Essential Oil
- Melissa Essential Oil
- Myrrh Essential Oil
- Palo Santo Essential Oil
- Peppermint Essential Oil
- Rosemary Essential Oil
- Sandalwood Essential Oil
- Sweet Orange Essential Oil
- Tea Tree Essential Oil
- Valerian Essential Oil

CHAPTER 5

Healing
Essential Oils

Essential oils are natural plant extracts that have been concentrated, usually using steam distillation. Most essential oils are derived from the leaves, roots, bark, flowers, and/or seeds of the plants from which they were obtained, though a few are made using whole plants. Essential oils are excellent for home remedies because they carry the concentrated healing power of plants; it often takes thousands of plants or plant parts to make a tiny bottle of essential oil.

Although approximately three hundred essential oils are commonly used by herbalists and naturopaths, many of these are fairly obscure and can be difficult to obtain. The most popular are listed in this chapter, and all are very easy to find at health food stores and online. Now that more people are using these oils for aromatherapy and home remedies, some large supermarkets and drugstores often carry popular essential oils, such as lavender and peppermint.

Many of these essential oils have a wide variety of uses. If you have a local store that will let you sniff and sample several oils, it's a great idea to pick a few whose fragrance you really enjoy, and then use this chapter to find all the ways you can use your favorites.

When shopping for essential oils, be sure to buy pure essential oils rather than those that have been mixed with other oils. Some terms to avoid include *fragrance oil* and *perfume oil*. These are normally scented products that are not suitable for therapeutic use. Though they smell nice, they don't have healing properties.

Because light has an adverse effect on potency, most quality essential oils are packaged in small bottles made of dark glass. When you get your essential oils home, be sure to store them in a cool, dark place to ensure they work the way you need them to.

If you are pregnant or nursing, talk with your obstetrician before using any essential oil. Some of these oils have the potential to cross the placental barrier and affect the fetus, while others have hormonal properties that can interfere with pregnancy. In addition, some essential oil should not be used on babies or children. Consult your pediatrician before using any essential oil with your child.

Take Note Some essential oils can cause irritation or reactions if they are applied at full strength to the skin, so they need to be diluted with carrier oils. A carrier oil is a vegetable oil, usually derived from seeds, kernels, or nuts. Carrier oils carry the essential oil onto the skin. Almond, avocado, olive, peanut, and pecan are some typical carrier oils. Stores that sell essential oils typically also sell carrier oils. Store your carrier oil with as much care as your essential oil.

Basil Essential Oil Ocimum basilicum

Basil essential oil has a clean, fresh scent and is an excellent natural anti-depressant. It promotes healthy digestion and has antiseptic, expectorant, and antibacterial properties.

BENEFITS

If you have a cold, you'll find basil essential oil wonderfully soothing. It is also effective in treating body aches and relaxing tired muscles, and it can alleviate pain and swelling associated with rheumatism. In addition, this essential oil is a natural insect repellent that can be used to soothe itchy bug bites.

HOW TO USE

Basil essential oil should be diluted with an equal amount of carrier oil before inhalation or topical use. If you plan to ingest it, simply blend it into water or add a drop or two to recipes that call for basil. For muscle aches, swelling, and minor pain, you can simply rub it into the affected area.

To ease cold symptoms, you can inhale it directly, diffuse it, or place a few drops into a hot bath and relax while inhaling the soothing vapors this essential oil produces.

TIPS AND PRECAUTIONS

Basil essential oil is safe for most people, but women who are pregnant should not use it as it is known to stimulate blood flow in the pelvic region. People with epilepsy should also avoid contact with it, as it may be one of many essential oils that provoke seizures.

Take Note An essential oil diffuser gently warms the oil to release its aroma into a room. Some use tea lights, where you place a few drops of the oil into some water, and then gently warm it over a candle. With electric diffusers, you place the oil on a pad or plate and an electric element warms it. A nebulizer converts the oil into microscopic particles and diffuses them throughout the room.

Chamomile Essential Oil Matricaria chamomilla

Sometimes referred to as blue chamomile essential oil or German chamomile essential oil, this powerful essential oil has a deep blue hue and a sweet, strongly herbaceous aroma. It has analgesic, anti-inflammatory, and anesthetic properties, and is useful as a decongestant and relaxant.

BENEFITS

The benefits of chamomile essential oil are many. It promotes rapid healing and soothes pain associated with bee stings, insect bites, and minor injuries, including bruises, strains, and sprains. In addition, it alleviates nervous tension, helps promote sound sleep, and can be used for natural stress relief.

HOW TO USE

Chamomile essential oil may be used undiluted. It is suitable for diffusion, direct inhalation, and topical application. It may also be ingested.

If you are suffering from a minor injury, you can simply massage a drop or two of chamomile essential oil into the affected area. If the skin is broken, apply it with a dropper and do not massage it; instead, just allow it to flow over the wound. You can use a cotton swab to dab up any excess.

To alleviate stress and promote better sleep, you can apply the essential oil to your pulse points. You can also add a drop or two to a cup of herbal tea and inhale the vapors while waiting for it to cool; then drink it while relaxing. Chamomile essential oil is also an excellent addition to soothing baths, and can be even more relaxing when combined with lavender essential oil.

TIPS AND PRECAUTIONS

Though opinions vary widely, because of chamomile's anti-inflammatory effects, women who are pregnant or breastfeeding may best avoid or use only very low doses of chamomile essential oil, chamomile tea, and other products that contain chamomile, as recommended by their doctor.

People who have sensitive skin or who are allergic to ragweed sometimes suffer irritation when exposed to this essential oil. If you notice itching, redness, or swelling developing, wash the affected area with soap and water immediately.

Clary Sage Essential Oil Salvia sclarea

Clary sage essential oil is highly prized for its antibacterial, antiseptic, and sedative properties. It is also an effective astringent that helps clear and calm problem skin.

BENEFITS

Among all essential oils, clary sage is one of the most effective for alleviating menstrual cramps and premenstrual symptoms. It also helps relieve insomnia, quiet busy minds, and promote rest and relaxation. In addition, clary sage essential oil uplifts the spirits and promotes clear, focused thinking.

HOW TO USE

Clary sage essential oil should be diluted with an equal amount of carrier oil before it is used in a diffuser or applied externally, but it may be directly inhaled. If you plan to use it as a dietary supplement, you can simply blend it with water and drink it.

To alleviate menstrual cramps and premenstrual symptoms, promote relaxation, and improve your overall mood, apply diluted clary sage essential oil to your pulse points and temples. Blend a drop or two into a cup of warm water or hot herbal tea and enjoy. You can also diffuse it in your home or office and inhale it directly.

TIPS AND PRECAUTIONS

Although clary sage essential oil is considered safe, it can cause skin irritation if applied undiluted. Small children should avoid contact with this essential oil. The International Federation of Professional Aromatherapists (IFPA) considers clary essential oil safe for topical use in low doses by pregnant women.

Eucalyptus Essential Oil Eucalyptus globulus

Eucalyptus essential oil has anti-infectious, antibacterial, antifungal, and antiseptic properties. It has a fresh, woody fragrance much like that of camphor.

BENEFITS

When inhaled, eucalyptus essential oil clears sinuses, eases coughs, and helps alleviate cold and flu symptoms. It can be applied topically to help combat ear inflammation, cleanse minor wounds, and reduce redness and pain associated with acne. It is also an effective ingredient for making natural insect repellent.

HOW TO USE

If you have cold or flu symptoms, the best way to use eucalyptus essential oil is to inhale it, either directly or by creating a steam bath with boiling water and a few drops of essential oil. You can also draw a hot bath and drip two drops of eucalyptus essential oil into it, soaking your body to relax and allowing the vapor to ease your congestion.

To treat minor wounds and alleviate redness associated with acne, dilute the essential oil with four parts of carrier oil and apply a small amount to the affected area.

TIPS AND PRECAUTIONS

While some essential oils may be applied full strength, eucalyptus essential oil should be applied only after dilution with a carrier oil.

Frankincense Essential Oil Boswellia carterii

Frankincense essential oil is prized for its balsamic, woody fragrance, and for its antifungal, anti-inflammatory, antiseptic, and sedative properties. It is also a natural expectorant and astringent.

BENEFITS

This fragrant essential oil combats infections, including strep throat. It is also useful for alleviating sore throats, calming coughs, and easing discomfort caused by pneumonia. It is a natural mood booster that alleviates stress and calms nervousness.

Why It Works Frankincense is derived from boswellia trees. Boswellic acid has properties found to inhibit growth of infected cells. University of Oklahoma studies point to the essential oil's ability to activate genes that suppress and kill human bladder cancer cells while ignoring healthy cells. Research is still restricted to the laboratory, but it provides support for frankincense oil's healing capabilities.

HOW TO USE

Frankincense essential oil must be diluted with an equal amount of carrier oil before being applied topically or diffused. It may be inhaled directly, and if you plan to use it as a dietary supplement, you can simply blend it with water.

If you are suffering from a cough, cold, flu, strep throat, or pneumonia, you can either diffuse the essential oil in your home or office, or you can apply it to your pulse points.

You can also add it to a hot bath and relax while inhaling its soothing vapors. The same methods may be used for easing nervous tension and alleviating stress. Increase its effects by blending a drop or two with a glass of water or herbal tea and drinking it.

TIPS AND PRECAUTIONS

Although frankincense essential oil is generally recognized as safe, it often causes skin irritation if applied undiluted.

Geranium Essential Oil Pelargonium graveolens

Geranium essential oil has a fresh, uplifting floral aroma. It has analgesic, antibacterial, and anti-inflammatory properties, and may be used as an effective diuretic. It is also a styptic agent that can help staunch bleeding from small wounds.

BENEFITS

This fragrant essential oil is a favorite with perfumeries, but its true value lies in its medicinal properties. It promotes healing, soothes insect bites and bee stings, relieves sore throats, and aids in alleviating fluid retention. Geranium essential oil can be used on burns, scrapes, and other minor wounds.

HOW TO USE

Geranium essential oil should be diluted with an equal amount of carrier oil before topical application or diffusion. To speed wound healing, simply apply a drop or two of diluted essential oil to the affected area, massaging lightly if skin is unbroken. The same remedy can be used for insect bites and minor rashes.

To relieve a sore throat or eliminate water retention, mix one or two drops of undiluted geranium essential oil in a glass of water or herbal tea and drink it.

TIPS AND PRECAUTIONS

Geranium contains the stimulant dimethylamylamine. Women who are in the first trimester of pregnancy should avoid contact with geranium essential oil, though it is considered safe to use topically in the second and third trimester. Also, it may cause skin irritation in sensitive individuals.

Take Note The use of essential oils during pregnancy continues to be a controversial topic, even among serious practitioners of aromatherapy. The International Federation of Professional Aromatherapists has published guidelines on this topic. Go to www.naha.org/explore-aromatherapy/safety#pregnancy for more information.

Ginger Essential Oil Zingiber officinale

Ginger essential oil is, of course, derived from fresh ginger root, which is also used for culinary and medicinal applications. Ginger essential oil has anti-inflammatory and anesthetic properties, and it is useful as a digestive aid.

BENEFITS

Like fresh ginger, ginger essential oil is useful for treating nausea, indigestion, and motion sickness. It is also an excellent treatment for soothing sore throats and easing congestion.

Why It Works Compounds in ginger help suppress prostaglandins, which are substances that control smooth muscle contractions, including those that can bring on intestinal cramping and contractions. The shogaol and gingerol in ginger also help those smooth muscles relax, alleviating painful symptoms of irritable bowel syndrome.

HOW TO USE

Dilute ginger essential oil by blending it with an equal amount of carrier oil before topical use. If you are planning to ingest it, you can simply blend it with water.

To soothe a sore throat or alleviate congestion, prepare a tea using boiling water and one or two drops of ginger essential oil. Blend it well and then inhale the vapors while waiting for the tea to cool enough to drink. Sip it slowly, making sure you coat the inside of your throat with the tea. You can also use this method for easing nausea, motion sickness, and indigestion.

TIPS AND PRECAUTIONS

Ginger essential oil is an anticoagulant and may enhance the effects of blood thinners, including warfarin, heparin, and aspirin. If you use blood thinners, be sure to talk with your doctor before using ginger essential oil.

Grapefruit Essential Oil Citrus paradisi

Grapefruit essential oil has a fresh, uplifting aroma that makes it effective as a mild antidepressant. It also has detoxifying, diuretic, stimulant, and cleansing properties.

BENEFITS

This sweet-smelling essential oil is a favorite not just because it is useful for brightening sour moods and combating depression but also because it is an effective headache remedy. It is also useful for easing water retention, clearing puffy skin, and promoting weight loss.

HOW TO USE

Grapefruit essential oil should be diluted with one part carrier oil prior to topical use. If you plan to ingest it, you can simply dilute it with water.

If you're retaining water and feel bloated, stir one or two drops of grapefruit essential oil into a glass of water and drink it. Repeat every few hours to maximize the diuretic effect. This same remedy works as an effective aid to weight loss, as does inhalation. If you are having food cravings, you'll find that this powerful remedy will usually stop them.

TIPS AND PRECAUTIONS

Grapefruit essential oil is toxic to cats. If your cat ingests it accidentally, contact your veterinarian right away.

Citrus essential oils can cause phototoxicity. If you have applied this essential oil to your skin, wait twenty-four hours before exposing that body part to direct sunlight.

Helichrysum Essential Oil Helichrysum italicum

Helichrysum essential oil is light yellow, with an earthy, fresh fragrance. It offers antimicrobial and antibacterial properties, and it is an effective diuretic, fever fighter, and expectorant.

BENEFITS

This essential oil is an excellent natural remedy for cold and flu symptoms. It can also be used to soothe minor pain from sprains and strains, and it is excellent for easing sore muscles. It may also be used to reduce the appearance of stretch marks and scars, and it can be applied to minor burns, cuts, and rashes to speed healing.

HOW TO USE

Helichrysum essential oil may be used without dilution. It is suitable for direct inhalation, topical application, and diffusion. If you plan to ingest it, mix it with water or herbal tea.

If you are suffering from a minor injury of any kind, you can simply apply helichrysum essential oil to the affected area and gently massage it in. Use the same technique when applying it to scars and stretch marks.

TIPS AND PRECAUTIONS

Although most people can use helichrysum essential oil with no side effects, those with sensitive skin may wish to dilute it with an equal amount of carrier oil before applying it to the skin.

Lavender Essential Oil Lavandula angustifolia

Lavender essential oil has a calming fragrance that promotes restful sleep. It also has analgesic, antiseptic, and antifungal properties.

BENEFITS

Lavender essential oil is a favorite for soothing nervous tension and easing insomnia. It can also be used to effectively halt premenstrual symptoms, reduce excessive oiliness on skin, and alleviate redness and swelling associated with acne. It is also useful for treating skin irritation and can help speed healing.

HOW TO USE

Lavender essential oil may be used without first being diluted. To promote restful sleep or soothe nervous tension, inhale it directly or apply one or two drops to your temples or to the pulse points on your inner wrists. These methods are also effective for combating premenstrual symptoms.

To alleviate oily skin, simply rub a few drops of lavender essential oil between your palms and apply it to the oily areas you wish to treat. To minimize pimples, dab a small amount of essential oil onto them with a cotton swab.

If you've got a minor rash, an insect bite, or a minor burn, scrape, or cut, drip a small amount of lavender essential oil onto the affected area and leave it there. Repeat the treatment as necessary.

TIPS AND PRECAUTIONS

Some individuals are sensitive to lavender essential oil and cannot apply it topically. Before using it on your skin, conduct a patch test by placing a small amount on the inside of your upper arm. If no rash develops within twelve to twenty-four hours, you can use it safely.

While many essential oils are safe for internal use, lavender essential oil can cause headaches, constipation, and other complications if ingested.

Lemon Essential Oil Citrus limonum

With its clean, fresh scent, lemon essential oil has the ability to brighten even the gloomiest mood. It also offers antibacterial, antifungal, antimicrobial, and anti-inflammatory properties, along with antiseptic, diuretic, and astringent qualities.

BENEFITS

Lemon essential oil is wonderful for use in cosmetic preparations. In addition, it is good for soothing indigestion and stopping food cravings as well as for taking the itch and sting out of insect bites.

HOW TO USE

This essential oil may be applied to skin without being diluted. It may also be inhaled directly, diffused, and ingested.

If you have oily skin, you can use lemon essential oil to promote balance by applying the essential oil to your skin and allowing it to remain there overnight. You can also smooth the appearance of wrinkles and stretch marks by applying a little lemon essential oil to them.

To treat insect bites, simply use a cotton swab to dab a small amount of lemon essential oil onto them.

Whether you are trying to stop food cravings or want to improve digestion, you can add one or two drops of lemon essential oil to a glass of water or a cup of herbal tea and drink it. Lemon essential oil is a mild diuretic, so you can use this remedy for alleviating water retention, too.

TIPS AND PRECAUTIONS

Be sure not to confuse lemon oil with lemon essential oil. Lemon oil is frequently sold for use as furniture polish and is not the same as lemon essential oil.

Lemon essential oil can be phototoxic, so be sure to wait twelve hours after it has been applied before exposing that area of skin to direct sunlight.

Melissa Essential Oil Melissa officinalis

Also known as lemon balm essential oil, Melissa essential oil has a fresh scent that is reminiscent of lemons. It has antibacterial, anti-inflammatory, anti-septic, and antiviral properties, and it is also an effective bactericide and sedative.

BENEFITS

Melissa essential oil is an excellent remedy for coughs and other cold symptoms. It may also help reduce fevers, and because it is a light sedative, it is perfect for use at bedtime. It is also useful for alleviating menstrual pain and stomach cramps, and it is good for soothing indigestion.

HOW TO USE

If you are suffering from cold symptoms, you can add one or two drops of Melissa essential oil to a cup of steaming hot tea and inhale the vapors before drinking the tea. You can also add a few drops to a hot bath and relax while enjoying the light, pleasant fragrance. The same remedy is useful for relieving pain associated with indigestion and menstrual cramps.

You can intensify the healing effects of inhaling vapor and drinking water or tea with Melissa essential oil by diffusing it in your home or office and by applying it to your pulse points.

TIPS AND PRECAUTIONS

Although Melissa essential oil is considered safe, it does sometimes cause irritation in individuals who have sensitive skin. If you notice redness or a rash developing, use warm, soapy water to remove the essential oil from the affected area.

Myrrh Essential Oil Commiphora myrrha

Myrrh essential oil has a wonderfully warm, earthy fragrance and a golden color. It has antifungal, anti-inflammatory, antiseptic, and antimicrobial properties as well as antiviral, astringent, and expectorant properties.

BENEFITS

This essential oil is highly prized for its ability to alleviate cold symptoms and soothe coughs, including those associated with bronchitis. It is also an effective treatment for athlete's foot and ringworm, and can reduce the appearance of stretch marks and wrinkles. It also alleviates pain associated with canker sores.

 Why It Works Myrrh oil contains terpenoids, chemicals with antioxidant and anti-inflammatory properties. Terpenoids are used in traditional medicine to treat a wide range of illnesses and diseases, and studies show that the ones found in myrrh oil may be useful in fighting infection, protecting against gum disease, and reducing inflammation and swelling.

HOW TO USE

Myrrh essential oil may be applied undiluted. If you are suffering from athlete's foot or a fungal infection such as ringworm, simply use a cotton swab to apply the essential oil to the affected area. Discard the cotton swab immediately after use. The same treatment can be used for canker sores.

If you'd like to use this essential oil on stretch marks or wrinkles, simply use a small amount on the affected area, rubbing it in gently and allowing it to remain overnight.

To soothe coughs and other cold symptoms, put two or three drops of myrrh essential oil into a diffuser and breathe deeply. You can also put a few drops into a hot bath and enjoy the fragrance while relaxing.

Myrrh essential oil is generally considered safe, and has been approved for use as a flavoring agent by the Food and Drug Administration.

Palo Santo Essential Oil Bursera graveolens

Palo santo essential oil has a sweet, slightly citrus aroma with strong woody notes. It has anti-infection, antiviral, anti-inflammatory, and antiseptic properties, and is also useful as a sedative and an immune system stimulant.

BENEFITS

This wonderful Peruvian essential oil is effective for relieving inflammation, muscle pain, and arthritis symptoms. It can also be used as a natural insect repellent.

HOW TO USE

Palo santo essential oil must be diluted with an equal amount of carrier oil before use. If you are suffering from muscle pain or inflammation, apply a few drops of diluted essential oil to the affected area and gently massage it into the skin.

To repel insects, you can apply it to your pulse points or make a mist by adding six drops of undiluted palo santo essential oil to ½ cup of water in a small spray bottle. Shake it thoroughly and spritz it on.

TIPS AND PRECAUTIONS

This essential oil should not be ingested. It sometimes causes skin irritation, so individuals with sensitive skin should watch for signs of redness and swelling. If this occurs, flush the affected area with carrier oil, wash the area with warm, soapy water, and then pat dry.

Peppermint Essential Oil Mentha piperita

Peppermint essential oil has a cool, clean aroma. It has analgesic, antibacterial, antiviral, and pain-relieving properties, and is useful as a digestive aid.

BENEFITS

Because it contains a high level of menthol, peppermint essential oil has a cooling, comforting effect that makes it ideal for soothing minor aches and pains, including tension headaches. It is useful for alleviating nausea and digestive discomfort. It can also help relieve itchiness and soothe eczema.

HOW TO USE

Peppermint essential oil must be blended with an equal part of carrier oil before it is applied to the skin or inhaled. If you plan to ingest it, you can simply blend it with water.

To ease pain or itchiness, apply diluted peppermint essential oil directly to the affected area and massage it in. If you are suffering from a tension headache, apply it to your temples and to the back of your neck. If you have a tendency to clench your jaw when stressed, you can also apply it to the area directly behind your ears to promote relaxation.

Peppermint essential oil can be used three different ways to alleviate nausea and improve digestion. You can inhale it directly, apply it to the bottoms of your feet, or mix one or two drops of undiluted essential oil into a glass of water or a cup of herbal tea and drink it. Drinking water mixed with peppermint is also an effective way to stop food cravings.

TIPS AND PRECAUTIONS

Peppermint essential oil burns the eyes, and also causes pain if it comes into contact with broken skin. If you accidentally get peppermint essential oil in your eyes or in other sensitive areas, do not use water to clean the area, as this will intensify the burning sensation. Flush the area with carrier oil instead and wait until the burning stops before washing with water.

Rosemary Essential Oil   Rosmarinus officinalis

Rosemary essential oil has a fresh, evergreen aroma that many people find wonderfully appealing. It has analgesic, antibacterial, fungicidal, and antiseptic properties and is an effective decongestant.

BENEFITS

Rosemary essential oil eases minor aches and pains when applied topically, and also helps improve circulation. This property also promotes healthy hair growth. If your skin tends to be oily, you can use rosemary essential oil to promote balance without causing moisture loss. You can also use it to relieve redness and swelling caused by acne. This essential oil is also excellent for promoting respiratory wellness. If you feel a cold coming on, you can use it to open your sinuses and ease minor chest congestion.

HOW TO USE

Rosemary essential oil does not have to be diluted before use. If you want to relieve muscle pain or cramping, apply a few drops topically and rub it into the affected area.

If you've got pimples, use a cotton swab to apply a small amount of essential oil to each one. Leave the oil on overnight and rinse it off in the morning. To promote healthy hair growth, add ten drops of rosemary essential oil to your favorite conditioner and blend well. Use the conditioner as you normally would.

If you'd like to use rosemary essential oil to promote respiratory wellness, there are a few ways to do so. It can be diffused, inhaled directly, or added to steaming hot water for inhalation. You can also add a few drops to a warm bath and inhale the vapors while relaxing.

TIPS AND PRECAUTIONS

While rosemary essential oil is made from the herb that is used in cooking, it can be toxic if ingested in large amounts. It is best for topical application and aromatherapeutic use.

Sandalwood Essential Oil Santalum album

Sandalwood essential oil has a sweet, woody fragrance that makes it a favorite in popular perfumes. It offers anti-inflammatory, anti-infection, antiseptic, and antiviral properties.

BENEFITS

If you have aging skin, acne, or scars, you'll find that sandalwood essential oil can greatly improve the appearance of your skin. When applied topically, it is also an effective remedy for treating hemorrhoids and cold sores. Sandalwood essential oil is also useful in easing bronchitis symptoms and promoting clear sinuses. Since it helps the body to produce melatonin, it promotes deep relaxation and is an effective natural sleep aid.

HOW TO USE

Sandalwood essential oil should be diluted with an equal amount of carrier oil before use. After diluting, apply it directly to the area of concern and allow it to remain on your skin.

If you are suffering from a cold or bronchitis, or if you wish to use this essential oil as a sleep aid, you can inhale it directly, apply it to your pulse points, or diffuse it in your home. You can also add a few drops to a warm bath and relax as you inhale its soothing vapors.

TIPS AND PRECAUTIONS

Sandalwood essential oil promotes sleep and does so quickly. Do not use it before driving or operating machinery.

Sweet Orange Essential Oil Citrus sinensis

Sweet orange essential oil has an uplifting fragrance that can help alleviate anxiety. It has antidepressant and sedative properties, and can be used to promote healthy circulation and improve digestion.

BENEFITS

Because it improves circulation, sweet orange essential oil is an excellent choice for topical use, particularly if you want to reduce the appearance of wrinkles and improve overall skin tone. It can also be used to combat water retention, relieve insomnia, ease nervous tension, and alleviate anxiety. Many women find it is an excellent essential oil for relief from menopause symptoms.

HOW TO USE

Sweet orange essential oil should be diluted with an equal amount of carrier oil before inhalation or topical use. If you plan to ingest it, you can simply mix it with water.

To improve skin tone, you can blend a drop of diluted essential oil with a small amount of your favorite moisturizer and apply it directly to your face. You can also blend two or three drops of diluted essential oil with your favorite body lotion and apply it to your arms, legs, hands, feet, and torso.

If you are feeling bloated, drink a glass of water with one or two drops of sweet orange essential oil mixed in. This makes an excellent replacement for artificially flavored drink powders and can help improve the taste of water so you'll stay hydrated.

To improve your mood, ease insomnia, and promote feelings of happiness, diffuse a few drops of diluted sweet orange essential oil in your home or office, or apply one drop of it to each of your temples or to the pulse points on the insides of your wrists.

TIPS AND PRECAUTIONS

Sweet orange essential oil is toxic to cats. If your cat accidentally swallows this essential oil, contact your veterinarian immediately.

Like other citrus essential oils, sweet orange essential oil can be photo-toxic. If you have applied it to your skin, wait twelve hours before direct exposure to sunlight. For this reason, it's best to apply skin tonics made with this essential oil before bedtime.

Tea Tree Essential Oil Melaleuca alternifolia

A pale yellow essential oil with an herbaceous, fresh aroma, tea tree essential oil offers valuable antimicrobial, antiseptic, and antiviral properties. It is also an effective bactericidal and antifungal agent.

BENEFITS

Tea tree essential oil is excellent for alleviating cold symptoms and clearing clogged sinuses. It is also useful for relieving irritated skin, clearing acne, and promoting rapid wound healing.

HOW TO USE

Like many other essential oils, tea tree oil must be diluted with an equal amount of carrier oil before it is applied to skin or diffused. It may be inhaled directly, and when used in baths and in steam treatments, it can be used without dilution.

If you have a cold or are suffering from allergies and have blocked sinuses, you can diffuse tea tree oil in your home or office to promote better breathing. You can also apply it to your pulse points, inhale it directly, or add it to a hot bath and relax while inhaling the vapors.

To treat acne, bug bites, and minor wounds, apply diluted tea tree oil to the affected area and allow it to remain there. Reapply as needed.

TIPS AND PRECAUTIONS

Tea tree essential oil is toxic to cats and dogs. If your pet accidentally swallows this essential oil, contact your veterinarian immediately.

Although tea tree oil is recognized as safe for humans, it can sometimes cause skin irritation. If you notice redness, swelling, itching, or hives, use carrier oil to remove it from your skin, and then wash the area with soap and water.

Valerian Essential Oil Valeriana officinalis

With a warm, slightly musky fragrance, valerian essential oil has bactericidal, diuretic, and hypnotic properties. It is often used as a sedative.

BENEFITS

Valerian essential oil is highly prized as a natural sleep aid. It is also effective for soothing restless legs syndrome, easing menstrual cramps, and alleviating hyperactivity.

Why It Works Research reported by the National Center for Biotechnology Information (NCBI) indicates valerian may be an effective sedative because it increases the neurotransmitter GABA (gamma-aminobutyric acid) between brain synapses. One study suggests valerian may allow GABA to be released from a nerve ending but stops it from returning, causing a sedative effect.

HOW TO USE

Valerian essential oil may be directly inhaled and diffused, and it can be applied to the skin without prior dilution. It may also be ingested. To improve its efficacy, use a combination of methods. Try blending one or two drops of valerian essential oil into a cup of herbal tea, inhaling the aroma, and sipping before bedtime. You can also add a few drops of essential oil to a hot bath, and you may apply the oil to your temples and pulse points, as well.

TIPS AND PRECAUTIONS

Valerian essential oil is a fairly strong sedative. Be sure not to use it before driving, operating machinery, or doing other tasks that require concentration.

PART III

EVERYDAY HOME REMEDIES

6 Common Ailments & Everyday Beauty and Body Care

7 Prenatal, Baby, and Child-Age Ailments

8 Everyday Wellness

9 Common Pet Ailments

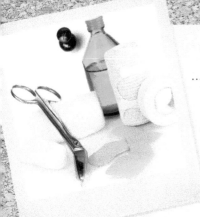

COMMON EVERYDAY AILMENTS

- Acid Reflux
- Anemia
- Arthritis
- Asthma
- Athlete's Foot
- Back Pain
- Boils
- Bruises
- Bunions
- Burns
- Bursitis
- Calluses and Corns
- Canker Sores
- Chafing
- Colds
- Cold Sores
- Colitis and Crohn's Disease
- Constipation
- Cough
- Cuts
- Diabetes
- Diarrhea
- Dry Eyes
- Dry Mouth
- Earache
- Eczema
- Eye Strain
- Fatigue
- Fever
- Fibromyalgia
- Flatulence
- Flu
- Gout
- Hangover
- Hay Fever
- Headache
- Heartburn
- Hemorrhoids
- Hiccups
- High Blood Pressure
- Hives and Itchy Skin
- Incontinence
- Indigestion
- Ingrown Toenail
- Insect Bites and Stings
- Insomnia
- Irritable Bowel Syndrome
- Kidney Stones
- Macular Degeneration
- Menopause Symptoms
- Menstrual Cramps
- Migraine
- Morning Sickness
- Motion Sickness
- Mouth Burns
- Muscle Cramps
- Nail Fungus
- Nausea
- Nosebleed
- Painful Gums
- Poison Ivy
- Premenstrual Syndrome (PMS)
- Receding Gums
- Restless Legs Syndrome
- Ringworm
- Scrapes
- Seasonal Allergies
- Sinus Pressure
- Sore Throat
- Spider Bites
- Splinter
- Sprain
- Sty
- Sunburn
- Swimmer's Ear
- Tick Bites
- Toothache
- Urinary Tract Infection
- Vaginal Dryness
- Varicose Veins
- Warts
- Water Retention
- Yeast Infection

CHAPTER 6

Common Everyday Ailments

If you're like just about everyone else on earth, you can name an ailment or two that you battle on a regular basis, whether it's a chronic issue or one that pops up in a specific season. These are nagging irritations you'd probably like to take care of quickly so you can go on with your normal activities in relative comfort.

The ailments listed in this chapter are chronic or occasional issues that you can address at home using everyday items and ingredients you have handy. If you are pregnant and experiencing any of the ailments listed in this chapter, check the Prenatal Ailments sections in chapter 7 for corresponding remedies that are safe for you to use. Also, do not use remedies that include essential oils on babies or children, or if you are pregnant. A few of the conditions listed here are more serious than an irritation, and we don't mean to imply they can be cured by a simple home remedy—rather, the remedies may offer relief from some of the symptoms you are experiencing. Once you've stocked your home with the necessary tools to combat the ailments in your family, you can provide quick relief for yourself, your spouse, your children, and even your pets (see Chapter 9).

You may be surprised at the simplicity of the ingredients and instructions for each ailment. We've provided at least three solutions to each, so if one doesn't quite work for you, you have more options before you schedule an appointment with your doctor. Chances are at least one of the remedies listed will provide you with some relief—and as these are generally based on foods, natural substances, and exercises or movement that you can do on your own, you can return to these remedies repeatedly for chronic conditions.

Acid Reflux

Acid reflux is also known as gastroesophageal reflux disease, or GERD. It happens when partially digested food, stomach acid, pancreatic juices, or bile travel upward from the digestive system into the esophagus, causing symptoms that include burning pain, coughing, nausea, and hoarseness.

EAT RAW ALMONDS

Raw almonds increase the digestive system's alkalinity, helping to neutralize some of the acid in your stomach. Eat a handful each day to bring your body's pH into balance.

EAT AN APPLE

Several substances can exacerbate acid reflux problems. These include greasy, fatty, and spicy foods, chocolate, nicotine, alcohol, and caffeine. If you can't avoid these substances, eat an apple after ingesting them. The fiber and pectin it contains absorb excess acid and help prevent acid reflux flare-ups.

DRINK BAKING SODA SOLUTION

Mix a tablespoon of baking soda with four ounces of water, stirring well so the baking soda dissolves. Drink it rapidly for quick relief.

Why It Works Baking soda is the common name for sodium bicarbonate. If you remember your high school chemistry, baking soda is a base—so, it neutralizes the acid in your stomach and esophagus. Use sodium bicarbonate sparingly; sodium is salt, which in high quantities can create other health issues.

When to See a Doctor When your heartburn is so severe that your throat hurts when you swallow food or pills, or your heartburn is accompanied by nausea and vomiting, see a doctor. Acid reflux that interferes with your daily lifestyle can be a symptom of a serious medical condition.

Anemia

Anemia develops when your blood lacks enough healthy red blood cells or hemoglobin. Hemoglobin is the protein in red blood cells that carries oxygen. If you are anemic, the cells in your body will not get enough oxygen. This typically causes feelings of weakness and exhaustion. Iron deficiency is the most common type of anemia. Other contributing factors include vitamin B_{12} deficiency, along with deficiencies in vitamin B_6, folic acid, or copper. If home remedies do not help alleviate symptoms of anemia, see your doctor to rule out other serious underlying causes.

COOK FOOD IN CAST-IRON COOKWARE

Cast-iron cookware (not the enamel-clad kind) helps significantly increase the iron content of the foods you prepare, helping to stop anemia symptoms by building strong, healthy blood cells.

TAKE A COMPLETE MULTIVITAMIN WITH IRON

Choose a high-quality multivitamin supplement and take the manufacturer's recommended dosage daily. Look for a supplement that contains B vitamins, folic acid, copper, iron, and vitamin C. Do not take more than the recommended dose with the idea that you are increasing the body's vitamin levels immediately; this can lead to indigestion and other complications.

KICK THE CAFFEINE

Kick your coffee habit and avoid drinking black tea as well, because caffeine can decrease iron absorption. Antacids also reduce the body's ability to absorb iron, so avoid them as much as possible.

Arthritis

Arthritis is a common joint disorder involving inflammation and pain. There are several types of arthritis, and severe cases often require medical intervention. If you have mild arthritis, home remedies may be enough to keep you comfortable.

GLUCOSAMINE SULFATE

Taking 1,500 mg of glucosamine sulfate—a naturally occurring compound in the fluid around the joints in the body—once a day has been found to help alleviate arthritis pain. Be careful not to get glucosamine hydrochloride, however, as this compound is not effective. Natural Medicines Comprehensive Database calls glucosamine sulfate "likely effective"—its second-highest rating—in treating arthritis pain. Studies show that taking the entire dose at once results in the body absorbing this compound more completely than splitting the dose.

Why It Works Taking glucosamine sulfate may increase the fluid surrounding joints and help thicken cartilage worn thin by osteoarthritis. It also may help prevent the breakdown of cartilage and joint fluid. In particular, the body needs sulfate to produce cartilage, so glucosamine supplements containing sulfate are more effective than those without it.

BROMELAIN FROM PINEAPPLE

Bromelain is an enzyme found in pineapple and has been used for hundreds of years in Central and South America to reduce inflammation. While there are only small amounts of the enzyme in a serving of the fruit, a more concentrated amount of bromelain is available in pill form, including a brand called Phlogenzym. Phlogenzym contains two other natural substances, rutosid and trypsin, that join with bromelain to work on joint pain. Clinical trials involving patients with arthritis have shown that this combination of enzymes and proteins can be just as effective as ibuprofen in reducing inflammation and relieving pain. Because the enzyme increases the risk of bleeding, though, it is not recommended for those on blood thinners or before surgery. Those who have allergies to pineapple, latex, wheat, or grass should consult their doctor before taking the enzyme.

APPLY FROZEN PEAS

A bag of frozen peas makes an excellent ice pack that conforms very well to small or irregular areas of the body, such as the hands. Lay a soft cloth between your skin and the bag of frozen peas, and leave the bag in place for fifteen to twenty minutes. You can use the same bag of peas over and over.

DRINK GINGER TEA

Ginger contains healing compounds that help reduce inflammation. If you drink ginger tea at least three times a day, you may notice that your arthritis symptoms are less pronounced. Be sure to choose a brand that contains natural ginger rather than artificial flavorings.

Asthma

Asthma attacks occur when tiny internal lung structures called bronchi and bronchioles come into contact with foreign invaders that are asthma triggers. These may include dust mites, mold, pollen, and pet dander, but in some cases, allergic reactions to foods and other substances can cause asthma attacks. Non-allergic asthma can be triggered by smoke (including secondhand smoke), strong perfume, exercise, dry or cold air, stressful situations and intense emotions, and even hearty laughter. Virtually all asthma patients carry a rescue inhaler to alleviate airway constriction—and home remedies should be used in conjunction with the inhaler, not in place of it. If home remedies and your inhaler do not alleviate symptoms, see your doctor immediately. Asthma can lead to lung damage.

DRINK COFFEE

Caffeine can open airways and help to dissipate asthma symptoms, something that doctors have known for nearly 150 years. The longstanding recommendation is three cups of strong coffee for an adult.

Why It Works Caffeine is closely related to another stimulant, theophylline, which has been used for many decades to treat respiratory illness. If you can't stand the taste of coffee, try black tea or Mountain Dew, though both contain about half the amount of caffeine.

TAKE DEEP BREATHS

Breathing slowly, regularly, and deeply when you feel an asthma attack coming on can help to calm symptoms. Get away from the asthma trigger before you begin. Sitting comfortably, blow your nose to clear it of any foreign matter. Now, inhale slowly through your nose, feeling the air moving as far into your lungs as possible. Exhale slowly, allowing your abdomen to relax as air exits your nasal passages. You can practice the same deep breathing exercise daily to strengthen your lungs.

EAT A SPICY PEPPER

Hot chili peppers and hot sauce contain capsaicin, which is a natural anti-inflammatory that can help you breathe easier. When you feel an asthma attack beginning, eat a few slices of pickled jalapeño pepper, a spoonful of hot salsa, or a spoonful of hot sauce. The spicier the pepper, the faster your symptoms will dissipate.

Athlete's Foot

Athlete's foot is caused by a fungus and is also called *tinea pedis*. It is a contagious infection that spreads easily from one person to the next, and is characterized by extremely itchy skin, sometimes with cracking and noticeable sores.

DRY IT UP

The fungus that causes athlete's foot thrives in moist places. No matter which remedy or remedies you try, be sure to keep your feet dry in between treatments. Keep your shoes and socks dry, too, and never wear the same socks for more than one day.

SOAK YOUR FEET IN VINEGAR

Vinegar kills foot fungus. Fill a footbath or a large pan with equal parts warm water and white vinegar. Leave your feet in the footbath for thirty minutes; then dry them well, dust them with foot powder, and put on a clean, dry pair of socks.

○ **Why It Works** Vinegar is made of acetic acid and water. Used primarily in cooking today, it once had many medical and industrial uses. In February 2010, the Journal of Food Protection published research that determined vinegar served as an antimicrobial, killing a range of microorganisms.

TRY A BORAX SOAK

A borax foot soak is simple to prepare. Fill a foot tub or washbasin with two gallons of hot water. Add ½ cup of borax powder and stir until the powder has dissolved. Soak your feet for ten minutes; then rinse them and pat them dry with a towel. You can add a few drops of your favorite essential oil to the footbath for a pleasant scent—some favorites include lavender, peppermint, and eucalyptus.

SWAB ON MOUTHWASH

To kill foot fungus, including athlete's foot, you can either use a cotton swab or cotton ball to apply small amounts of mouthwash to the area around your toenails and between your toes three times daily for about a week, or you can speed up the process by soaking your feet in a footbath or basin filled with an inch of mouthwash and warm water to cover the affected area. If you have a bad case of foot fungus, expect a little stinging. Try to keep your feet in the footbath for five minutes. In most cases, a single foot soak is all it takes to eradicate athlete's foot; toenail fungus usually requires multiple treatments.

SPRAY ON PEROXIDE

Eliminate foot fungus by spraying your feet with a hydrogen peroxide solution made with 50 percent water and 50 percent hydrogen peroxide twice daily. Be sure to get in between your toes and around your toenails, since these areas serve as hiding places for fungi.

WEAR SHOES

If you use public showers such as those at the gym, be sure to wear shower shoes at all times. Never expose your bare feet to damp surfaces in public places.

Back Pain

Back pain can be the result of an injury, or it can be due to a chronic condition involving bones, tendons, muscles, and/or ligaments. It's important to have all back injuries checked by a physician before deciding to use home remedies, since an untreated injury can get worse and eventually leave you debilitated. Home remedies are best for minor back pain, such as stiffness from sitting too long, soreness from working out, standing on your feet longer than usual, peripheral pain associated with pregnancy, or even just poor posture.

TURMERIC

The University of Maryland Medical Center suggests that ingesting 300 mg of turmeric three times a day can be effective for alleviating back pain. You can buy turmeric in pill form, or use it (albeit in smaller amounts) in your food—the spice is one of several used in Indian curries. Do not use turmeric as a supplement if you're on a blood-thinning medication, as it may increase the effects of the medication.

MASSAGE WITH MINT

Peppermint essential oil contains menthol that soothes soreness and promotes relaxation. Apply the peppermint oil directly to the skin and work it in using deep circular motions. If your pain is in an area that's difficult for you to reach, ask someone to help you with this task. As an added benefit, the scent of peppermint oil promotes overall relaxation, which may also help to ease your pain.

HEAL WITH HEAT

Heat helps sore muscles relax, easing pain and increasing circulation, which in turn promotes healing. Use a hot water bottle or a heating pad, either lying on your stomach or sitting comfortably with the heat source firmly pressed against the affected area. Spend at least fifteen minutes using heat therapy three times a day. If you use an electric heating pad, be sure not to fall asleep while it is in use.

When to See a Doctor If your back pain is only one of a complex of symptoms that include numbness in your legs, lethargy, tingling, or urinary incontinence, you may have a serious medical condition. This may also be true if the pain is so intense that you struggle to stand up.

Boils

Boils are deep skin abscesses surrounded by red, swollen skin, and almost all of them have yellow or white pus-filled centers. Most boils are caused by bacteria that have penetrated the skin's surface. Although these abscesses can be extremely painful and unpleasant to look at, with proper treatment and patience they can heal in two to three weeks. It is important to note that some boils need medical treatment. If you have a fever, fatigue, or swollen lymph nodes in conjunction with a boil, seek medical attention.

USE A HOT COMPRESS

A hot compress made with a soft cloth and very hot water increases circulation and will speed up the natural healing process. Apply the compress every few hours. The boil should open and drain on its own. Do not squeeze it or attempt to open it with needles or other implements.

TAKE A BATH IN EPSOM SALT

Epsom salt helps speed boil draining and can also help soothe localized pain associated with a boil. Draw a comfortably hot bath and add one cup of Epsom salt. Stir the salt with your hand to dissolve it before getting into the tub. Soak yourself until the water cools. Repeat this twice a day until your boil heals.

SOOTHE WITH HONEY

After your boil bursts, wash the area thoroughly and coat it with honey. Let the honey dry and then cover it with a clean cloth to protect the area but still allow it to breathe.

Bruises

Bruises are caused by trauma to the delicate tissues and blood vessels that lie just beneath the skin's surface. They can be caused by blunt force, pinch injuries, and even excessive rubbing and chafing.

MASSAGE WITH CASTOR OIL

Castor oil was once a popular remedy for many ailments; sometimes it worked, and sometimes it didn't. One of the best uses for castor oil—one that actually works—is as a remedy for bruises. Apply a small amount to the skin covering the bruise and massage it in to help reduce swelling and speed healing.

Why It Works The oil from the castor bean plant has the ability to increase the flow of lymph in your body, allowing lymphocyte cells—integral parts of the immune system—to remove toxins from the injured tissues. This process speeds healing.

STOP SHINERS WITH SUGAR

Applying sugar to an area that has just suffered an injury can help reduce the size of bruises, and in some cases, it can prevent bruising altogether. Wet a cloth with water, dip it into sugar, and massage the area for thirty seconds to a minute.

MASSAGE WITH MOUTHWASH

Minimize the appearance and duration of bruises by massaging the affected area with mouthwash shortly after the injury takes place. Spend a few minutes working the mouthwash into the skin, massaging lightly to prevent further injury to capillaries.

Bunions

A bunion is a red, swollen, bony lump that forms at the base of the big toe, where it joins the foot. They are sometimes caused by years of wearing shoes that chafe and pinch.

CHECK YOUR SHOE SIZE

One of the most common causes of bunions is wearing shoes that are too small. You may not realize that your feet continue to grow throughout your adult life, so the shoe size you had in your twenties can be as much as a size and a half too small when you're in your forties. Buying shoes that fit can take the pressure off your toes, which in turn relaxes your foot into a position that will not cause a bunion. Visit a shoe store where a professional can measure your foot properly.

TRY AN ASPIRIN FOOT SOAK

Although the best remedy for bunions is to wear comfortable shoes that do not place pressure on the injured area, irritation can occur after bunions have developed. One of the best ways to stop the pain is to treat your feet to an aspirin soak. Fill a footbath or basin with warm water. Crush six adult aspirin tablets and allow the resulting powder to dissolve in the footbath. Soak your feet until the water cools.

RICE IS NICE

Fill a clean sock with rice, tie a knot in the end of it, and place it in the microwave for one minute to ninety seconds, or until it is hot. Place the heated sock on your sore bunion and leave it there until the rice has cooled. You can reuse the same sock as often as you like.

Burns

A burn occurs when the skin has been damaged by a heat source or a caustic chemical. Treatment varies, depending on the severity of the burn; home remedies are suitable only for first-degree burns that do not burn all the way through the outer layer of the skin.

COOL WITH YOGURT

Cold yogurt straight from the refrigerator will help to soothe the pain associated with a minor burn. Cover the burn with a thin layer of yogurt and leave it in place for fifteen minutes. Rinse the area with cold water afterward.

USE YELLOW MUSTARD

Yellow mustard is another soothing remedy for minor burns, and can even help prevent blisters. Cover the affected area with mustard, leaving it in place for at least fifteen minutes. Wash the burn with cool water after the treatment.

TEA TREE OIL COOLS BURNS

After you have administered the basic first aid for burns—running cold water over the burned area for at least ten minutes—applying a few drops of tea tree oil can cool a minor burn and help reduce the pain. Be careful with the oil, as it is toxic when swallowed.

Why It Works According to the American Cancer Society, laboratory experiments show tea tree oil works as a topical antiseptic for several bacterial infections and on germs resistant to certain antibiotics. Although the oil has been used in the United States only since the 1980s, it has been used by Australian physicians since the 1920s.

Bursitis

The painful condition known as bursitis is actually an inflammation of a fluid sac called the bursa, which is found inside a joint. This often chronic condition can take a very long time to heal. Doctors usually prescribe over-the-counter painkillers like ibuprofen or a prescription-strength NSAID. Use of these painkillers over a long period can cause stomach upset, and may even lead to ulcers.

BROMELAIN FROM PINEAPPLE

Bromelain is an enzyme found in the stem and juice of a pineapple. The enzyme's anti-inflammatory properties make it helpful for both arthritis and bursitis sufferers. In fact, the University of Maryland Medical Center lists bromelain as complementary therapy for bursitis, and states that taking 250 mg twice a day reduces inflammation. Taken in recommended amounts, the supplement is considered safe, but consult your doctor before taking the enzyme if you are allergic to pineapple, latex, wheat, or grass, and if you are on blood thinners, or prior to surgery.

THE YELLOW SPICE

Turmeric, the yellow spice that gives Indian curries their pungency, contains an active ingredient called curcumin that is well known in both Western and Eastern medicine for its medicinal capabilities. Laboratory research has shown that curcumin has the ability to target inflammation, reducing the pain and soreness in muscles and joints. Daily doses are shown to be safe over as long as a three-month period. You can buy cur-cumin in pill form, which is probably the easiest way to take enough of it to have the desired effect.

Why It Works Curcumin is the reason for turmeric's positive health effects. It's a pleiotropic type of molecule, capable of interacting with molecules that cause inflammation and preventing them from creating swelling and pain. Clinical trials are in progress to determine if curcumin may be a viable treatment for certain cancers.

COLD AND HOT

Ice the afflicted joint for ten to fifteen minutes at a time for several days, until the swelling and inflammation has subsided. Follow this with a soothing heating pad for fifteen or twenty minutes at a time. The heat will help stimulate circulation and restore your flexibility over time.

Calluses and Corns

Calluses are areas of thick, hardened dead skin that have formed to pro-tect the skin from pressure and friction. They can eventually become thick and even painful. Corns are simply calluses that form where the toes rub together. They can eventually become thick and even painful.

SOFTEN WITH CORN SYRUP

Corn syrup is ideal for softening corns, making it easier to scrub them away. Cover the corn with a thick layer of corn syrup and then cover it with a bandage. Keep reapplying corn syrup and a bandage after every shower or bath, and your corn will eventually shrink as the hardened tis-sue softens.

DISSOLVE WITH VINEGAR

Vinegar contains acetic acid, which helps soften and dissolve painful corns. Before going to bed, soak a cotton ball in vinegar. Secure it to your corn with a bandage and then cover the bandage with plastic wrap to keep the vinegar from dripping. Wear thick socks to bed. In the morning, remove the sock, the plastic wrap, the bandage, and the cotton ball. Repeat each night. Your corn will slowly dissolve.

TRY AN ASPIRIN PASTE

To soften calluses using aspirin, crush six adult aspirin tablets and place them in a small bowl. Add ½ teaspoon of warm water and ½ teaspoon of lemon juice to create a paste. Rub the paste onto the calluses and cover the area with plastic wrap. After the callus softens, you can use a pumice stone to rub the dead skin away.

SOAK IN PEROXIDE

To soften calluses on your feet, prepare a footbath with a gallon of hot water and one cup of hydrogen peroxide. Soak your feet for up to thirty minutes; then dry them and buff them with an exfoliator. Apply thick lotion and put on a pair of heavy socks. Leave the socks in place until all the lotion has been absorbed to prevent messes and to ensure that you don't slip on hard-surfaced floors.

When to See a Doctor If you have diabetes or another condition that diminishes blood circulation in your feet, do not treat calluses on your own. Peeling away the dead skin can lead to ulcers and infection when you have diabetes. Have your feet cared for by a podiatrist.

Canker Sores

Canker sores are small, shallow sores located on the inside of the mouth. They often appear as red circles surrounded by white, slightly raised rings.

APPLY A TEABAG

Black tea contains tannins, which soothe inflammation and can help relieve pain. Brew a cup of plain black tea and then pull the teabag out of the cup and allow it to cool. Press the cool teabag to the canker sore, leaving it in place for approximately five minutes. After the tea has cooled, drink it plain or with a small amount of honey. Repeat this treatment two to three times a day until the canker sore heals.

SOOTHE WITH AN ANTACID TABLET

Antacid tablets contain calcium carbonate, which neutralizes acid that causes canker sores to hurt. Simply place an antacid tablet in your mouth, using your tongue to press it against the canker sore. Leave it in place until it dissolves. You can repeat this process up to three times a day.

CHECK YOUR TOOTHPASTE

Scientists in Norway recently completed a study that linked sodium lauryl sulfate (SLS), a common ingredient in toothpaste, to canker sores in users. If your toothpaste has SLS and you get frequent canker sores, try switching to one that doesn't have it.

Chafing

Chafing is caused by skin that rubs uncomfortably against other body parts or clothing that is too tight or misaligned. Chafed skin is often quite irritated and tender, and in many cases it is also swollen. Be sure to wear breathable clothing made with natural fibers and check the affected area frequently to ensure that it stays protected.

EASE WITH CORNSTARCH

Use cornstarch to create a barrier between areas of skin that tend to rub up against one another. Apply the cornstarch after showering and thoroughly drying your skin; this will prevent friction and help heal chafed areas.

HEAL WITH CALENDULA OIL

The oil from this plant in the marigold family has performed well in pharmacological studies, showing real antiviral and anti-inflammatory properties that make it an important additive in topical medicinal ointments and oils. You can purchase it as an essential oil and use it directly on your chafed area to reduce inflammation and soothe your skin. (Watch for allergic reactions, and don't use it if you're pregnant, as calendula oil may trigger increased blood flow. The oil is also believed to interfere with conception, although this effect is not proven.)

SOOTHE WITH DIAPER RASH OINTMENT

Serious cases of chafing cause broken skin that can sometimes bleed. Diaper rash ointment helps to soothe and lubricate chafed skin while discouraging worse irritation.

Chicken Skin

Also known as keratosis pilaris (KP), chicken skin consists of tiny plugged hair follicles that can be exacerbated by dry winter air. The condition usually affects the upper arms and the thighs.

BUFF WITH A PUFF

Before showering, apply a light moisturizer to the affected area and buff it lightly with a polyester bath puff. After showering, use more moisturizer to soften the skin. This remedy may be repeated daily until your skin is smooth. Be sure to clean the bath puff between uses.

DISSOLVE WITH APPLE CIDER VINEGAR

The acid in apple cider vinegar can dissolve the hardened skin that's clogging the hair follicles on your arms and legs. Before showering, apply a thin layer of apple cider vinegar to the affected area with a cotton pad. Wait fifteen minutes, and then shower, scrubbing the area you just treated with a polyester bath puff and moisturizing soap. Repeat the treatment every other day until your skin is smooth.

COCONUT OIL IN THE SHOWER

It's sold for cooking, but so is cider vinegar so why not try coconut oil for your KP? The nearly solid oil comes in screw-top jars making it easy to get a few fingers full of the stuff to apply in the shower. Once it comes in contact with the heat of your hand, the solid oil liquefies and goes on easily. Your skin will absorb it quickly, and most people find the coconut scent fairly subtle.

Colds

Despite all of the discoveries in modern medicine and the eradication of many diseases, there is still no cure for the common cold. The cold is a tough nut to crack, mainly because it doesn't come from just one virus—in fact, hundreds of different viruses can cause a cold. The best we can hope for today is to shorten the duration and relieve the symptoms of any cold we contract.

CHICKEN SOUP COULDN'T HURT

Since Maimonides first recommended chicken soup for a cold back in the 1100s, mothers have been dishing up this "Jewish penicillin" to their sick children. Don't get the powdered varieties—it's got to be real chicken soup, cooked from a chicken, to have the desired effect. The soup will thin the mucus in the nasal passages and chest, and it may even block some of the viral activity that clogs up the sinuses.

Why It Works Mount Sinai Medical Center did the lab research on chicken soup. They found that cysteine, an amino acid found in chicken (and also found in other high-protein foods), acts on the lungs the way a drug called acetylcysteine does—as a powerful decongestant for phlegm.

GRATED FRESH GINGER

Ginger tea is one of the great natural remedies, with positive results for dozens of ailments. When you've got to clear your head of a miserable cold, however, you want more than a spicy teabag—you want to bring out the big guns, so to speak. Peel about an inch-long piece of fresh ginger root, and grate it directly into your cup. Add eight ounces of boiling water. Steep it for ten minutes, and then strain out the ginger root. Add some cayenne or jalapeño pepper if you want more bite and an anti-congestive effect, though you may not need it.

YOGURT: CREAMY PREVENTION

With all of the benefits of eating probiotic yogurt, perhaps it should not be a surprise that a study published in the *British Journal of Nutrition* in found that two specific probiotics, LGG and BB-12, reduced the duration and severity of colds in 200 college students. The scientists believe that the probiotics work because they reduce the immune system's reaction to the cold virus, making colds shorter and less debilitating. Grab a cup of yogurt with active probiotic cultures every day, and keep colds at bay.

Cold Sores

Also known as fever blisters, cold sores are caused by the type 1 herpes simplex virus. They occur near the mouth and, when left untreated, can cause serious pain and itching. If you have a cold sore, avoid touching other parts of your body before washing your hands, because the virus can spread. Do not kiss another person or use items someone else might use.

To help protect others from coming in contact with the virus, wash cups, glasses, and silverware that you have used immediately after finishing a drink or meal. If home remedies do not seem to be helping, seek medical attention. Though generally considered to be a sexually transmitted disease, some strains of herpes can be contracted via indirect contact.

SPEED HEALING WITH WITCH HAZEL

Itching, tingling sensations often precede cold sore formation. As soon as you suspect you have a cold sore forming, apply witch hazel with a cotton swab. Repeat this treatment twice daily to reduce cold sore size and promote rapid healing.

PROMOTE HEALING WITH PEPPERMINT

Peppermint essential oil has powerful antiviral properties that help keep cold sores from becoming larger. Use a cotton swab to apply a few drops of peppermint essential oil to the affected area, repeating twice a day until the cold sore is gone.

Why It Works In laboratory studies, peppermint has been shown effective against the herpes simplex virus type 1 and 2, which is related to the virus in cold sores. Used topically, it can help to defeat one-time or recurring cold sores.

RUB ON ALCOHOL

You can shrink and soothe itchy cold sores by dabbing them with a cotton swab that has been dipped in rubbing alcohol. Brace yourself, because this remedy does sting for a moment. Because cold sores are contagious, be sure to wash and disinfect your hands after touching them.

PRACTICE PREVENTION

If you are prone to cold sores, prevention is just as helpful as topical remedies. Stress, reduced immunity caused by cold or flu, fatigue, and poor dietary habits can increase the likelihood of an outbreak. Take good care of yourself by exercising to reduce stress, eating a healthful diet based primarily on whole plant foods to increase immunity, and making rest and relaxation a priority in your daily life.

Colitis and Crohn's Disease

Colitis and Crohn's disease are inflammatory diseases of the gastrointestinal system that require a doctor's care. But even with the help of a specialist, they cannot be cured. Crohn's disease is particularly insidious, because it can attack any part of the digestive system, from the mouth to the anus—and this condition can be even more infuriating because doctors don't know why it happens. Medical treatments can be aggressive, so any kind of natural alternative can be good news for patients.

THE PINEAPPLE EFFECT

Have you ever wondered why fresh or frozen pineapple can't be used in Jell-O? Bromelain, an enzyme found in pineapple, breaks down the proteins in the gelatin and turns the dessert into a bowl of glop. This ability made bromelain a topic of greater scientific study, leading to the discovery that bromelain can thwart diseases that inflame the bowel. How much pineapple you should eat remains to be seen, but if you want a concentrated effect, try the supplements in pill form.

MACAROONS CALM INTESTINES

Coconut has long been known as a digestive aid, calming many an upset stomach and irritated bowel. You can buy a bag of shredded coconut and eat a couple of tablespoons a day, but many people choose macaroons (which are naturally gluten-free) to help chase away the effects of colitis and other bowel afflictions. Two a day seems to be the recommended dose.

Why It Works Coconut contains medium-chain triglycerides, or fatty acids, that are absorbed in the digestive tract more easily than long-chain triglycerides like soy, corn, and vegetable oil. Studies in the United Kingdom and Spain found that medium-chain triglycerides also help with the body's ability to absorb nutrients.

CUT DOWN ON DAIRY

People with colitis or Crohn's disease often find that dairy products cause gas, bloating, abdominal pain, and diarrhea. These are all symptoms of lactose intolerance. Limiting dairy products—in particular, milk, processed and creamy cheeses, butter, and ice cream—can bring relief from these symptoms. Switching to lactose-free products helps, as well, while allowing you to retain the nutritional benefits of dairy foods.

Constipation

Constipation is characterized by bowel movements that are difficult to pass, which can cause real discomfort. When you finally do manage to have a bowel movement, your stools are typically dry and dark. Constipation can be caused by a number of issues that are simple to change: too little fiber or water in your diet, not enough exercise, or certain kinds of medicines that you take for blood pressure, pain relief, depression, iron deficiency, or several other seemingly unrelated conditions. Pregnancy can also bring about constipation. If you are pregnant and constipated, turn to Prenatal Ailments in chapter 7 for remedies that are safe to use.

DRINK A CUP OF COFFEE

Because coffee contains caffeine, which stimulates bowel movements, it is one of the best remedies for constipation. If you don't like coffee, choose another beverage that contains caffeine—black tea, green tea, and even caffeinated soft drinks. Wait thirty minutes, and if you still haven't had a bowel movement, have another beverage. Repeat this remedy up to four times. However, remember that heavy caffeine use on a daily basis can cause unpleasant side effects such as insomnia. After this episode of constipation has been resolved, focus on preventive diet and exercise habits to eliminate future discomfort.

MORE WATER AND FIBER

Increasing the amount of fiber in your diet gives your intestines the material needed to push digested and undigested food through your system. Fruits, vegetables, and whole grains are all excellent sources of fiber—and they're all good for you anyway. Increasing the amount of water in your diet provides lubrication to your intestines, as well, allowing your body to do what comes naturally.

TAKE CASTOR OIL

As it turns out, great-grandma was right to prescribe castor oil for constipation. Though this remedy is vile-tasting, it is an effective laxative. Take two tablespoons of castor oil, swallowing them down without food or water. Give the oil about thirty minutes to make its way into your system before eating or drinking anything. You can chew a piece of gum to get rid of the taste, if you like. The oil should cause a bowel movement within six to twelve hours. *Pregnant women should not take castor oil. Do not take castor oil if one of your symptoms is abdominal pain.*

DRINK EPSOM SALT

Combine two teaspoons of Epsom salt with eight ounces of water. Stir it until the Epsom salt has dissolved completely and then add lemon juice to increase palatability, if you like. Drink the mixture down as rapidly as you can and then stay in the vicinity of a restroom until you have a bowel movement. In most cases, this laxative works within thirty minutes; in some cases, it can take several hours to work. If four hours pass and you still haven't had a bowel movement, repeat the treatment. Do not take more than two doses of Epsom salt in a twenty-four hour span, and be sure to consult a physician if the remedy fails to work the second time around.

When to See a Doctor In severe cases, failure to pass stools leads to bowel obstruction, which can be life threatening. It's also possible that a tumor in your intestine is preventing normal bowel movement. If you experience constipation for three weeks and home remedies don't work, see your doctor.

Cough

Coughing is your body's way of removing irritants from the lungs. While productive coughs that are removing excess mucous from the airway are important to allow, dry, irritating coughs can cause discomfort and hoarseness. If a cough doesn't clear up in a week, see your doctor to be sure it is not a symptom of a serious ailment.

DRINK GINGER TEA

Ginger has antihistamine and decongestant capabilities that have made it a staple of Eastern medicine for centuries. To soothe a cough and alleviate accompanying throat pain, brew a cup of ginger tea, either with a teabag that contains real ginger or with two drops of ginger essential oil. Breathe the soothing vapors as you wait for the tea to cool; then drink it. Repeat this treatment every three hours.

TRY THYME TEA

Thyme is a well-known treatment for coughs, bronchitis, and upper respiratory infections. You may find its ability to relax your throat muscles and reduce inflammation to be effective for you, too. Steep two teaspoons of crushed thyme leaves—from your garden or from the herb and spice shelf in your favorite supermarket—in a cup of boiling water for ten minutes. Strain, add some honey and lemon if you like, and drink.

COAT YOUR THROAT WITH HONEY

Honey is a sweet, soothing remedy for dry, irritating coughs. Simply swallow a tablespoon of honey. Wait fifteen to thirty minutes before you eat or drink anything, so the honey has time to soothe irritated throat tissues.

Cuts

Little nicks and cuts can easily be treated at home. If a cut is deep or won't stop bleeding, you may need stitches; in that case, see your doctor or visit an urgent care center.

DAB WITH CORNSTARCH

Its moisture-absorbing properties make cornstarch good for staunching the bleeding from minor cuts and scrapes. Place a little bit directly on the cut and the bleeding will stop.

SPEED HEALING WITH VITAMIN E

After washing and drying a superficial cut, you can snip a hole in a capsule of vitamin E and pour the contents onto the cut. Repeat this every twelve hours until the cut has healed. Be sure to wash the affected area before each treatment.

Why It Works Vitamin E is the most abundant antioxidant in the human skin, but ingested vitamin E can take seven days to benefit the skin. Applying vitamin E topically speeds this substance to where it's needed. Avoid UV light (sunlight) after application, as it destroys this vitamin.

PREVENT INFECTION WITH HONEY

Honey is a natural antibiotic that speeds healing and that can help prevent infections. Apply a dab of honey to a fresh cut and cover it with an adhesive bandage. Repeat the treatment every twelve hours until the cut has healed. Be sure to wash the affected area before each treatment.

Diabetes

When your body can't process insulin—a hormone that carries glucose (sugar)—it can't function properly, and the result is the condition we know as diabetes. If you have this disease, either the pancreas can't produce insulin (type 1), or the body can't respond to the insulin it produces (type 2), but either problem results in a cascade failure of other systems if it's not treated under a physician's supervision. Not every case of diabetes requires insulin injections and daily monitoring of blood sugar levels, but the majority of those with the disease do need these precautions.

No home remedy can substitute for a doctor's care. However, some remedies do assist in controlling blood sugar levels and preventing them from rising precipitously after a meal.

CINNAMON IN CAPSULES

Research has revealed that cinnamon can help control blood sugar—but not the cinnamon you use on oatmeal and in cookies. Spice-rack cinnamon contains coumarin, which the body can't tolerate in high doses (it causes liver damage). Instead of doling out teaspoons of potentially harmful cinnamon from a shaker, pick up high-quality cinnamon pills at your favorite nutritional supplement store. These pills are not regulated by the FDA, but they may help you control your sugar levels.

A SPOONFUL OF VINEGAR . . .

. . . helps the sugar go down? Indeed it does, according to a study completed at Tokyo University. Subjects who took two teaspoons of vinegar daily for twelve weeks experienced decreases in hemoglobin A1C, a red blood cell involved in blood sugar control.

Why It Works Acetic acid—what makes vinegar taste so sour—inhibits the activity of some enzymes that digest carbohydrates. When vinegar is in the intestines, it allows some sugars and starches to pass through undigested. These sugars and starches then have no impact on blood sugar.

THE POWER OF FENUGREEK

Well known in India as a cooking spice, the aromatic fenugreek plant produces tiny seeds in long pods. These seeds can be used whole or ground into a powder, either of which has been shown to lower blood sugar in clinical trials. Researchers in India found that adding 100 g of fenugreek seed powder to the diets of patients with type 1 diabetes reduced their fasting blood glucose levels, lowered total cholesterol and triglycerides, and improved their glucose tolerance.

Diarrhea

Diarrhea is often caused by a viral or bacterial infection, and involves the discharge of loose, watery stools.

EAT COCONUT

Treat yourself to two heaping tablespoons of coconut, either on its own or mixed into a cup of vanilla yogurt. Repeat six hours later if the diarrhea has not stopped.

DRINK APPLE CIDER VINEGAR

If harmful bacteria is the culprit, apple cider vinegar will often eliminate it. Stir two tablespoons of apple cider vinegar into a glass of water and drink it. Repeat six hours later if the diarrhea has not stopped.

TRY PINK BISMUTH

While pink bismuth has many uses, treating diarrhea is the one it is actually marketed for. And it does work. Follow the directions on the bottle, in liquid or pill form.

EAT YOGURT

Yogurt with live, active cultures can help reset your digestive system and bring your stomach and intestines back into normal functioning. The cultures are actually bacteria—the good kind, called "probiotics"—that help process food through your digestive tract. If the diarrhea you're experiencing comes from using antibiotics, yogurt can be the fastest way to replace the good bacteria that antibiotics kill along with the bad. Check the package to be sure your yogurt has live cultures—many of the highly processed brands retain the taste of yogurt without the living cultures.

When to See a Doctor If diarrhea persists past three days or is accompanied by vomiting, fever, and chills, you may have food poisoning. These symptoms may also signal something more serious, and can lead to dehydration. Call your doctor if diarrhea continues beyond a thirty-six-hour virus.

Dry Eyes

Dry eyes are often caused by dry air, though they sometimes occur when you have been working at a computer or watching television without blinking for a long period of time. This uncomfortable condition prevents your eyes from removing debris. Dry eyes can also cause dizziness, vertigo, and a feeling akin to motion sickness.

USE A HUMIDIFIER

If you think dry air is causing your discomfort, the best treatment is to add moisture to the atmosphere. Using a humidifier will help, especially if you have central heating and air-conditioning.

COVER WITH CUCUMBER

If you believe eye strain is the cause of your dry, tired eyes, cut two thin slices of cucumber, lie down comfortably, close your eyes, and cover them with the cucumber slices. Stay in this position for twenty minutes. Listen to soothing music or an audio book if you feel bored or unproductive.

Why It Works Cucumbers contain antioxidants believed to reduce swelling and irritation—under the eyes and anywhere on your body. Though cucumber's effect on puffy eyes has yet to be studied, barring an allergy to cucumber, this remedy is harmless. A cold pack may be equally effective.

ARTIFICIAL TEARS

A number of manufacturers make eye drops that temporarily replace the moisture your eyes are not producing on their own. These "artificial tears" contain an ocular lubricant, bringing immediate relief for eyes that are dry from staring at a computer screen for too many hours. Eye drops that relieve redness or bring allergy relief are not effective for dry eyes, so be sure you've selected drops that lubricate the eyes.

When to See a Doctor When dry eyes are common, or your eyes are irritated, red, and tired on a daily basis, it's time to see your ophthalmologist—particularly if you have stringy mucus in your eyes, light sensitivity, or blurred vision. Medical conditions and medications may be responsible.

Dry Mouth

Dry mouth occurs when the mouth fails to produce enough saliva to keep mouth tissues adequately lubricated. This problem can make eating, talking, and swallowing difficult, and it can contribute to peripheral problems such as cracked skin and bad breath. This is often a problem for older adults as well as for people who take antihistamines, allergy medications, antidepressants, beta-blockers, high blood pressure medications, and a number of other medications. Dry mouth is also common for people undergoing cancer treatment, or for diabetics. Ensure that you're drinking enough water to keep your body lubricated—sixty-four ounces of water a day—and if you still need help, try the following remedies.

CHEW SUGARLESS GUM

Sugarless gum helps increase saliva production and alleviate the discomfort caused by dry mouth. Chew it as often as you like, enjoying a fresh piece when the flavor begins to dissipate.

DRINK LEMON JUICE

Lemon juice promotes salivation and can rapidly reverse dry mouth. Mix one tablespoon of fresh lemon juice with a tablespoon of water and drink it.

USE A DRY MOUTH TOOTHPASTE AND MOUTHWASH

A mouthwash and toothpaste formulated to help with dry mouth can kill the bacteria that can form in your mouth when there's not enough saliva to wash them away at normal intervals. These products do not cure dry mouth, but they can ease the symptoms and help you maintain a healthy mouth, protecting your gums and teeth as well.

Why It Works Products made for dry mouth are formulated to match the pH range of normal saliva, helping to guard against the harmful bacteria. They also contain no alcohol, the germicide found in most mouthwashes, which can also act as a drying agent.

INCREASE HUMIDITY

Dry air can cause problems with dry mouth. Use a humidifier to keep air comfortably humid. For rapid relief, take a hot shower after drinking a glass of water.

Earache

Earaches can be caused by infection, or they can be caused by sinus pressure. They can also be caused by excess moisture trapped inside the ear. If your earache worsens or does not seem to be getting better after two days, contact your doctor. You may need antibiotics. For more remedies to lessen the pain of ear infections, see the entry in chapter 7 under child ailments—remedies that work for children also can have a positive effect for adults.

SOOTHE PAIN WITH A BLOW DRYER

To relieve pain and ensure that there is no moisture causing complications inside your ears, turn your blow dryer on low and aim it at your ear, holding it about twelve inches away from your head. Stop after thirty seconds or if your ear becomes hot and uncomfortable.

WARMTH AND VINEGAR

The combination of heat and a vinegar/alcohol solution is a tried-and-true method recommended by doctors for decades.

1. Mix equal parts of white vinegar and isopropyl (rubbing) alcohol.
2. Lie down on your side, and use an eyedropper to place a couple of drops of the solution into your ear.
3. Place a warm compress or heating pad over your ear (not *in* your ear), and allow the heat to work its way in.
4. Wait about ten minutes.
5. Place a cotton ball or pad on the outside of the affected ear, and stand up. Allow the liquid to drain out of your ear into the cotton ball.

KILL BACTERIA WITH VODKA

To kill the bacteria that may be causing your ear to hurt, fill an eyedropper with vodka. Lie on your side and drip the vodka into your ear. Remain in this position for ten minutes while the vodka does its work; then stand up and drain your ear into the sink or into a clean towel. If you don't have vodka, you can use rubbing alcohol for this treatment.

Eczema

When you get itchy, reddened patches on your skin for no apparent reason, you mostly likely have eczema. This term actually refers to a group of skin conditions that seem to occur in people who have other sensitivities and allergies, including seasonal allergies, hay fever, and asthma. Eczema can be caused by any number of triggers: a new laundry detergent, a soap in a new scent, getting overheated or being too cold, being sick with a cold or flu, wearing something rough or itchy, coming into contact with pet dander, or prolonged stress.

SENSITIVE SKIN PRODUCTS

Liquid soaps, shampoos, and skin lotions that say they are for "sensitive skin" are useful for people with eczema. These are often unscented, or the scents and other ingredients they contain are less likely to irritate your skin than normal products.

MOISTURIZE WITH CERAMIDES

Choose a moisturizer or lotion that contains ceramides, a fatty compound that should already be in your skin. People with eczema often have lower than normal levels of ceramides in their skin. Replacing these compounds can help with the itching and redness.

SOOTHE WITH CHAMOMILE

Steep dried chamomile in a cup of boiling water for fifteen minutes or longer. Don't drink it (you can, but it won't be as effective); instead, soak a piece of gauze in the tea and apply it to the eczema patch on your skin. Leave it there for twenty minutes. You can do this repeatedly throughout the day if you like, until the inflammation subsides.

Why It Works Chamomile has natural anti-inflammatory properties that reduce swelling, itching, and redness. The flower contains terpenoids, which give the plant its scent and have antibacterial properties, and flavonoids. These properties have demonstrated anti-inflammatory and anti-allergic properties during in vitro laboratory studies.

Eye Strain

Eye strain usually happens when you keep your focus on one thing, such as a television, computer screen, or book, for long periods of time, or drive long distances without taking sufficient breaks. Because eye muscles are often overtired and strained, puffiness sometimes occurs in the eye area.

TRY TEABAGS

Brew a cup of tea with two teabags in it, preferably black tea or orange pekoe tea. Remove the teabags and allow them to cool; then lie down and place them over your eyes. Leave them in place until they have cooled completely. The caffeine in the tea helps to promote circulation and ease eye strain, while the warmth of the teabags helps tired eye muscles relax.

SHIFT YOUR FOCUS

When you are working at your computer for a long time, take frequent breaks to focus on a distant object and stretch your body. Follow the twenty-twenty-twenty rule: Every twenty minutes, give your eyes a break by looking at an object twenty feet away from you for twenty seconds. In addition, take a fifteen-minute break at least every two hours. You can also position your chair so that your eyes are level with the upper edge of the computer screen. This helps alleviate glare, plus it helps your eyes remain relaxed.

SOOTHING MASSAGE

Here is a tip from the Mayo Clinic: Massaging the muscles over your brow, temple, and upper cheek can help reduce the discomfort of eye strain.

1. Using your bare fingers, massage your upper eyelid against your brow bone. Do this for about 10 seconds.
2. Next, gently massage your lower eyelid against the bone below your eye, also for 10 seconds.

This technique not only will help relax the muscles around the eye but also may stimulate your tear glands, getting them to produce the moisture your eyes need.

Fatigue

Fatigue is caused by a lack of sleep, often compounded by stress and life's daily pressures. Poor nutrition and dehydration can make it worse. If you believe you get enough sleep and are eating a healthful diet, constant fatigue could be a symptom of an underlying health problem.

SWITCH TO TEA

While coffee and black tea both contain caffeine that can temporarily perk you up, tea also contains L-theanine, an amino acid that helps increase the body's production of serotonin, dopamine, and gamma-aminobutyric acid, three neurotransmitters that help eliminate fatigue. Enjoy your tea hot or iced, with or without your favorite sweetener.

INHALE PEPPERMINT ESSENTIAL OIL

Peppermint essential oil stimulates the brain and promotes mental stamina. Apply a few drops of peppermint essential oil to a cotton ball and place it near the area where you are working or relaxing, inhaling deeply every few minutes. You can also place the essential oil in a diffuser and enjoy its effects in your home or office.

EAT AN EGG

Now that eggs have been removed from the "enemy" foods list, we can rely on them once again for their sound nutritional value and high protein content. Both of these attributes make the vitamin-rich egg one of our best tools to fight fatigue and a number of other stress-related ailments. The vitamin A, iron, riboflavin, and folic acid content of eggs makes them a potent energy booster. Keep a few hard-boiled eggs in the refrigerator for midafternoon pick-me-ups.

When to See a Doctor Chronic fatigue is a medical condition and easily overlooked because of its diverse symptoms. Tiredness throughout the day is also a symptom of sleep apnea, a breathing disorder that disrupts sleep—often without you knowing it. Specialists can diagnose these conditions and other causes of fatigue.

Fever

Fevers usually signify that your body is in the process of fighting an infection, which is why they so often happen in conjunction with colds and the flu. If your fever rises above 103°F and worsens or does not break, you may have a serious infection that requires medical intervention. Consider a fever like this an emergency, and contact your doctor immediately.

DRINK GINGER TEA

Hot ginger tea can help induce sweating and break your fever. Prepare a strong cup of ginger tea, either with teabags that contain real ginger, or with fresh grated ginger. You can even make yourself a cup of herbal tea and add two drops of ginger essential oil. Inhale the aroma as you wait for the tea to cool; then drink it. Repeat every two to three hours to promote healing.

COOL IT WITH ICE

When you're suffering from a fever or are very hot, drink a beverage with ice to help bring your body temperature down. At the same time, apply ice packs to the back of your neck and your inner arms to help cool the blood. Leave the ice packs in place for just a few minutes at a time, repeating the treatment every ten minutes or so until you are more comfortable.

TAKE A HOT BATH

If your fever is below 103°F, take a hot bath, which will trick your body into reducing its temperature. If you are not in the mood for a bath, use a hot compress on your forehead instead. If your fever is 103°F, use a cool compress or take a cool shower to help keep your temperature down.

Fibromyalgia

Fibromyalgia causes pain in your soft tissues, morning stiffness, overall fatigue, and restlessness when you're trying to sleep. If you're already frustrated by the diagnosis of this painful condition and your doctor's view that it's a psychosomatic illness, it may be time to try some home remedies.

FRANKINCENSE FOR INFLAMMATION

In Ayurveda medicine, frankincense (derived from the genus *Boswellia*) is used to combat inflammatory conditions like arthritis and fibromyalgia. You can purchase frankincense extract in your favorite health food store. If you're already taking ibuprofen or other anti-inflammatory medications, frankincense may decrease their effectiveness—be sure to check with your doctor before adding this to your treatment regimen.

TART CHERRY JUICE

The nutrients in tart cherries have been found to work as disease-fighting agents, as a safeguard against carcinogens, and as a cholesterol-lowering food. They also have anti-inflammatory properties. Drink an 8-ounce glass of tart cherry juice daily, and more during a flare-up of your fibromyalgia.

Why It Works Red fruits and vegetables contain anthocyanins, antioxidants that fight disease. These nutrients encourage healthy circulation, keep your nerves functioning properly, and even have some cancer-fighting abilities.

Flatulence

Flatulence now and then is natural—in fact, doctors say that we normally pass gas fourteen to twenty-three times a day—but in some cases, excessive gas can cause embarrassment and discomfort. Flatulence is usually caused by exposure to unfamiliar foods that are hard for the body to digest.

EAT YOGURT

If you are often plagued by flatulence, you may not have enough beneficial bacteria in your gut. These bacteria are responsible for breaking down fibrous food for complete digestion. Choose yogurt with live, active cultures, and eat a cup of it every day for at least a week to recolonize beneficial bacteria.

DRINK PEPPERMINT TEA

If your flatulence has been caused by dietary indiscretion, you'll find that drinking a cup of hot peppermint tea can quickly solve the problem. Brew a strong cup of peppermint tea, either with a teabag or with two or three drops of peppermint essential oil. Repeat the treatment in three hours if gas persists.

TALK A WALK

That gassy, bloated feeling you get after eating some foods (like a bean burrito) is as much from improper digestion as it is from the food's fiber content. Taking a walk can help ease the digestive process, encouraging what you've consumed to keep moving through your system.

When to See a Doctor If eating dairy products causes your flatulence, you may be lactose intolerant—meaning your body has trouble digesting the sugar in dairy. Taking an enzyme called lactase before you eat dairy can help. Your doctor can help you test for this fairly common condition.

Flu

Influenza, usually referred to simply as the flu, is a viral infection that attacks the upper respiratory system and sometimes involves the lungs. If you are suffering from the flu and it doesn't improve after five days, seek medical attention.

EAT CHICKEN SOUP

Your mom was right when she told you to eat chicken soup every time you came down with the flu. The combination of piping hot liquid and nutrients in the chicken broth help to soothe symptoms and prevent excessive mucus from forming. Only real chicken soup will work; broth made with bullion is not as effective.

EASE CONGESTION WITH EUCALYPTUS ESSENTIAL OIL

To ease congestion, place a towel on your kitchen table. Put a large bowl on top of the towel and fill it with boiling water. Add three drops of eucalyptus essential oil, sit down in a chair, place your head over the bowl, and cover your head with a second towel. Inhale the vapors, breathing deeply and emerging for fresh air if your face feels too hot. Keep a box of tissues close by so that you can pause to blow your nose as congestion clears.

TRY HELICHRYSUM ESSENTIAL OIL

Helichrysum essential oil can help alleviate cold and flu symptoms in a variety of ways. You can inhale it directly if you wish, but you may find it more effective to apply it to your pulse points or diffuse it in your home or office. You may also add a few drops to a hot bath and relax while inhaling its soothing vapors, and you can add one or two drops to herbal tea, inhaling the vapors as you wait for it to cool.

Why It Works Helichrysum essential oil contains sesquiterpene hydrocarbons that assist in reducing inflammation. These compounds may reduce the swelling of nasal passages that typify the flu. Neryl acetate, a monoterpenoid contained in the oil, relaxes tension in the tissues.

When to See a Doctor Most of us will recover from the flu in a week or so without medication, but a number of people are at risk for serious complications from this illness. If you are a senior citizen, if you have a pulmonary (breathing) or heart condition, or if your baby is afflicted with the flu, see a doctor right away. People die of the flu every year, and they are most often in one of these categories.

Gout

The mention of gout may bring to mind images of Henry VIII walking stiffly with a cane, but gout is very much a 21st-century condition as well. It comes from an overabundance of uric acid crystals that leave the blood and move into the joints, most often in the toes. Gout is terribly painful, and no one who has had it wants to have it again. Lifestyle changes will help keep it away.

SOUR CHERRIES FOR GOUT

A recent study showed that eating sour cherries could diminish the likelihood of a gout attack. The exact number of cherries may differ from one individual to another, but a study by the Boston University Medical Center found that eating at least ten cherries a day was enough to do the trick.

Why It Works According to the study published in *Arthritis and Rheumatism*, cherries block the reabsorption of uric acid and help redirect urate into the urine, where it can be excreted. Cherries may reduce production of uric acid by blocking xanthine oxidase, an enzyme used to make uric acid.

LIMIT ALCOHOL INTAKE

Excessive use of alcohol—more than two drinks a day—can significantly increase the possibility of gout. Take it easy at happy hour and limit the after-dinner drinks.

PREVENT THE NEXT ATTACK

Once you have had gout, it's time to look at dietary changes that will help to keep you from having it again. Many foods contribute to the excess uric acid in your system. Limit the amount of these foods to keep uric acid at bay: red meat, dried beans, anchovies, fish, asparagus, mushrooms, spinach, yeast (used in bread), gravy, and shellfish. Salt also increases uric acid, and fructose (as in high fructose corn syrup) is the only carbohydrate that increases the body's supply of uric acid.

Hangover

Nausea, a splitting headache, dehydration, and an overwhelming feeling of fatigue are all signs of hangover, which is caused by drinking too much alcohol. When you have a hangover, you may also feel dizzy, be sensitive to light, and have difficulty concentrating.

DRINK GINGER TEA WITH HONEY

Hangover symptoms are worsened by dehydration and low blood sugar. Ginger, one of the magic bullets of homeopathic remedies, can be particularly helpful for a hangover because of its well-documented ability to alleviate some kinds of nausea. Don't use more than 1 g of ginger in a single day, however, to avoid heartburn or irritation of the soft tissues in your mouth.

1. Prepare a cup of strong ginger tea with teabags that contain real ginger, or use 2 or 3 drops of ginger essential oil blended with hot water.
2. Stir 1 tablespoon of honey into the tea and breathe the vapors while waiting for it to cool.
3. Drink the tea.
4. Have a second cup in 30 minutes to 1 hour, and keep on drinking fluids until you begin to feel human again.

Why It Works Ginger slows down biochemical pathways in much the same way that aspirin and ibuprofen do, and it promotes circulation in the same way that these painkillers can. Chemicals called gingerols and shogaols relax the intestines, relieving nausea, vomiting, cramps, and other digestive upsets.

EAT CHICKEN SOUP

After your nausea subsides, have some chicken soup. The nutrients in the soup will help revitalize you and start the digestive process. If you're feeling brave, add crackers to your soup or have some plain toast with it.

AN OUNCE OF PREVENTION . . .

You've heard it before, the best way to avoid a hangover is to abstain from drinking alcohol. But there are other ways to keep a hangover at bay, or at least lessen the effects of a hangover and still imbibe on occasion. Try to drink in moderation, and stop drinking when you start to feel tipsy. Keep yourself hydrated by alternating your alcoholic drinks with a glass of water. Don't drink on an empty stomach. Eating foods that will "soak up" the alcohol, such as bread and even fish is often helpful. You can also try drinking Pedialyte before going out clubbing. It will provide your body with some of the electrolytes it loses during overuse of alcohol, thus reducing hangover symptoms.

Hay Fever

Hay fever is usually brought on by exposure to airborne seeds and pollen. Symptoms include teary, itchy eyes, an itchy throat, a runny nose, and sneezing that won't stop. The best way to begin treating yourself for hay fever is to minimize exposure to the pollen and seeds. Anti-allergy remedies can help, as can some surprisingly simple remedies.

DRINK A CUP OF COFFEE

Coffee contains a natural antihistamine that helps alleviate hay fever symptoms. You can enjoy it hot or iced, but be aware that adding dairy products can stimulate mucus production, so lighten it with a nondairy creamer, if needed. Be sure to drink plenty of non-caffeinated beverages throughout the day, since coffee is a diuretic and even mild dehydration can lead to increased congestion.

HAVE SOME GARLIC

Garlic is a natural antibiotic that boosts the immune system, and it contains a substance called allicin, which helps relieve congestion by thinning mucus. Enjoy a dish such as pasta, soup, or stew made with plenty of garlic.

TRY A NETI POT

Nasal irrigation has become a top recommendation of ear, nose, and throat physicians and surgeons, first to clear out congestion and crusts in the nasal passages, and then to rinse away some of the irritants than cause these symptoms. You can purchase a neti pot—a teapot-like device that makes it fairly easy to pour water through your sinuses—at most pharmacies. The irrigation process works by helping the hairlike cilia inside your nose and sinuses work properly, pushing mucus out of the way of your breathing passages.

1. Mix 1 pint of lukewarm, sterilized (previously boiled) or distilled water with 1 teaspoon of salt.
2. Fill the neti pot with the solution.
3. Position your head over the sink at a 45-degree angle.
4. Align the spout of the neti pot with your top nostril, and pour the solution through that nostril.
5. The solution will flow through your sinuses and out the other nostril.
6. When you've poured all the solution through, blow your nose to remove any remaining liquid.
7. Refill the neti pot and repeat the process on the other side.
8. When you're finished, rinse out the neti pot and let it air-dry.
9. Repeat these steps once a day until the symptoms of hay fever finally pass, or the allergy season ends.

Headache

The brain does not have pain receptors, but the muscles, arteries, nerves, skull, subcutaneous structures, eyes, ears, mucous membranes, and sinuses in the head and neck can all ache. Headaches happen when any of the head's sensitive regions are disturbed, often by tension, pressure, dehydration, or changes in blood pressure. There are more than two hundred specific types of headaches. For remedies specific to migraine, see Migraine later in this chapter.

EAT ALMONDS OR CASHEWS

Magnesium is an excellent headache remedy because it relaxes the blood vessels, arteries, and muscles. Many nuts are an excellent source of magnesium. An ounce of almonds has 80 mg, and an ounce of cashews contains 75 mg. Peanuts and peanut butter contain less but may still make a difference; peanuts have 50 mg of magnesium per ounce, and two tablespoons of peanut butter provide the same amount of magnesium.

APPLY MENTHOL RUB

Pungent menthol rub is a remarkable headache remedy. When applied to the temples, forehead, and back of the neck, it first stimulates nerves and then prompts them to relax. You can achieve the same effect by dabbing peppermint essential oil, which also contains a high level of menthol, on your head's sensitive regions.

Why It Works Menthol, a naturally occurring compound found in peppermint or cornmint, has an ability to trigger cold-sensitive receptors in the skin. This creates the penetrating cool sensation that becomes such a potent pain and congestion reliever.

PEPPERMINT COMPRESS

Make peppermint compresses by steeping three peppermint teabags in two cups of hot water for about five minutes. Squeeze the teabags to remove all the liquid from them, and then add ice to the water. Dip a soft cloth in the liquid and apply it to your aching head.

Heartburn

Heartburn actually has nothing to do with the heart, but is an uncomfortable burning sensation below the breastbone caused by stomach acid irritating the esophagus. Too much food in the stomach or too much pressure on the stomach can cause acid from the stomach to seep into the esophagus. Foods high in fats and oils may also lead to heartburn.

EAT AN APPLE

"An apple a day keeps the doctor away" was a slogan for a marketing scheme back in the early 1900s, and it turns out that there's truth to the old axiom after all. Apples neutralize excess acid in the stomach by creating an alkaline state, and just a few bites of a sweet apple (not the tart Granny Smith–type varieties) can prevent stomach acid from backing up into the esophagus. Try a Red Delicious, Honeycrisp, or Braeburn apple for this purpose.

DRINK PAPAYA JUICE

An eight-ounce glass of papaya juice contains enough of the enzyme papain to quell heartburn almost instantly. If you dislike the flavor of papaya juice or if it is unavailable in your area, you can take papaya extract tablets instead.

GO FOR GINGER

Candied ginger stops heartburn rapidly, prompting the muscles that push acid upward to relax. Simply chew and swallow a piece of candied ginger about the size of the tip of your thumb, and heartburn should fade within ten minutes. If you dislike candied ginger or have none on hand, you can drink a cup of strong ginger tea instead.

When to See a Doctor If none of these remedies work for you, and your acid reflux persists on a daily basis or wakes you at night, it's time to consult a doctor. Constant acid backup can cause ulcers in the esophagus and, over time, patients can have trouble swallowing.

Hemorrhoids

Hemorrhoids feel much worse than they are—an important thing to remember when you're in considerable pain. Each hemorrhoid is a swollen vein in the anal canal, and they can appear inside the canal or just outside the anus. Hemorrhoids come from too much pressure—i.e., pushing—on the anal walls. Additional remedies for hemorrhoids can be found in the Prenatal section of chapter 7, though the remedies listed here are considered safe for pregnant women to use, too.

KEEP IT CLEAN

Cleansing the area after each bowel movement can bring soothing relief as well as reduction in the inflammation. Pat—don't wipe—the anus with a medicated wipe or a pre-moistened baby wipe. If your hemorrhoids are particularly uncomfortable, take a sitz bath: Fill your tub with warm water deep enough to cover the anus when you sit down. Get into the tub and sit in the warm water for fifteen minutes. Repeat this as often as you like.

ICE IT DOWN

Fill a plastic resealable bag with ice, and wrap it in a small towel. Apply this cold pack to your anal region several times a day, for ten minutes each time. The cold will help reduce the swelling.

DRINK PRUNE JUICE

When you have hemorrhoids, the last thing you want to do is push hard to expel a bowel movement. Prunes and prune juice can help by bringing both fiber and lubrication to your intestines and by acting as a mild laxative. (If you hate prune juice, drinking water will help irrigate the intestines so you can move your bowels without straining.)

Why It Works Prunes and prune juice contain soluble and insoluble fiber, which draw water into your intestines, making stools softer and easy to pass. A 2010 study by the University of Iowa found prune juice was a more effective laxative than psyllium, a common ingredient in over-the-counter laxatives.

Hiccups

Hiccups are caused by intermittent muscle spasms in the diaphragm. These spasms can happen for a variety of reasons: sometimes you swallow air when you eat, sometimes carbonated beverages stimulate nerves that activate the diaphragm, and sometimes they seem to happen for no reason at all.

A SPOONFUL OF SUGAR

Swallowing a teaspoon of dry sugar often stops hiccups immediately. The feeling of the sugar in your mouth and throat temporarily interrupts the nerve signals that instruct the diaphragm to bounce up and down.

SUCK ON A LEMON

Sucking a slice of lemon is another way to interrupt nerve signals to the diaphragm. As the muscles in your mouth and throat react to its sour flavor, the body recalibrates and hiccups cease. If you have no fresh lemon, swallow a tablespoon of lemon juice or apple cider vinegar instead.

HOLD YOUR BREATH

It's an old-fashioned remedy, but it works in most cases of hiccups: Take a deep breath and hold it while you slowly count to ten. This increases the level of carbon dioxide in your blood, which recalibrates your breathing and stops the spasm of hiccups. If just holding your breath doesn't work, trying breathing inside a paper bag for thirty seconds.

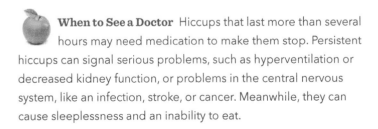 **When to See a Doctor** Hiccups that last more than several hours may need medication to make them stop. Persistent hiccups can signal serious problems, such as hyperventilation or decreased kidney function, or problems in the central nervous system, like an infection, stroke, or cancer. Meanwhile, they can cause sleeplessness and an inability to eat.

High Blood Pressure

High blood pressure is one of the most potentially destructive conditions a person can have. It can lead to heart attack, stroke, dementia, and kidney damage. Your doctor is likely to write a prescription to keep your blood pressure under control, but you can take action on your own to keep your blood pressure within the normal range.

BEET JUICE LOWERS BP

Research conducted in Australia revealed that beet juice can have an immediate impact on lowering blood pressure. The study showed that even a single glass of beet juice lowered systolic (the top number) blood pressure by four to five points within hours of drinking the juice.

Why It Works Beet juice supplies a high concentration of nitrates, which the body converts into nitric oxide. The new compound relaxes and dilates blood vessels, bringing the blood pressure down as blood flows more smoothly through the body. Leafy green vegetables also supply large amounts of nitrates.

THE DARK CHOCOLATE FACTOR

Eating a one-ounce square of dark chocolate with at least 70 percent cocoa brings flavonoids to the body that help to lower blood pressure. Note the one-ounce limit: If you start eating all the chocolate you can get your hands on, you will increase your weight and negate the benefits of the dark chocolate.

WALKING FOR HEALTH

You've heard it a thousand times: Eat less, exercise more, and you will improve your health. There's no question that regular exercise will help you keep your blood pressure down by burning calories, training your heart to work efficiently, and clearing plaque and cholesterol out of your arteries. Build thirty minutes into your day at least five times per week to start seeing and feeling the difference.

Hives and Itchy Skin

Hives are red, hot, itchy welts or bumps that raise up on the skin when connective tissues release a substance called histamine, which is the body's natural defense against allergens and irritants. People break out in hives for a variety of reasons. Often, it's because of something that has been eaten, but sometimes it is because of exposure to cold or sun. Stress and nervousness can cause hives, as can viral infections. The remedies here will help with hives and also with any itchy rash or patch of skin.

TAKE A HOT SHOWER

One of the fastest, easiest ways to eliminate itching is to take a hot shower, remaining in the water between fifteen and twenty minutes. This prompts the body to release all of its histamine, after which the itching will stop. It will take your body several hours to make more histamine.

DAB ON WITCH HAZEL

The astringent in witch hazel encourages blood vessels to contract and limits the amount of histamines the skin can produce. Pour a few drops of witch hazel onto a cotton ball and dab it onto the itchy area for instant cooling and relief.

COOL WITH ALOE VERA

After showering and drying your skin, apply a generous amount of aloe vera gel to the affected area. Reapply every four to six hours.

Why It Works Aloe vera has been known as a healing plant for centuries, but scientists only began to study its effects in 1973. Though researchers disagree on why the succulent works, they have found that aloe gel can heal open wounds, even wounds that have persisted for years.

PEPPERMINT COMPRESS

Make peppermint compresses by steeping three peppermint teabags in two cups of hot water for about five minutes. Squeeze the teabags to remove all the liquid from them, and then add ice to the water. Dip a soft cloth in the liquid and apply it to irritated skin.

Incontinence

Involuntary leakage from your bladder can have a negative impact on your social life, your ability to travel, and your overall comfort and sense of well-being. You can take steps at home to keep incontinence from becoming a factor in your quality of life, but you also should see your doctor to rule out any kind of urinary tract infection or issue that may be causing the problem.

SKIP THE TRIGGERS

Too much caffeine and alcohol can trigger bladder activity, and drinking liquids in the evening can lead to many sleep interruptions to use the bathroom during the night. Cut back on the coffee, tea, cola, or other caffeinated beverages, and try not to drink anything at all after the dinner hour.

Why It Works Caffeine is a natural diuretic—it increases the need to urinate. The more caffeine you ingest, the more time you'll spend in the bathroom. Alcohol also stimulates the bladder and serves as a diuretic. That's why there's often a line for the bathroom at parties.

KEGELS FOR CONTROL

Exercises to strengthen the pelvic muscles—called Kegel exercises, after the doctor who invented them—can help you guard against stress incontinence, the involuntary release of urine when you sneeze, cough, or laugh. Talk to your gynecologist or proctologist about the correct way to do Kegel exercises.

ASIAN HERB BLEND

Gosha-jinki-gan is a compound made from a blend of ten specific herbs. The supplement has shown promise in a study of forty-four women in Japan. The women in the study had decreased frequency of urination and a higher quality of life after taking 7.5 g of gosha-jinki-gan daily. While such a small study can't be considered conclusive evidence, the herb blend shows promise.

Indigestion

Indigestion usually happens after a heavy meal, because you've overloaded your system and your stomach is having difficulty handling its contents. Though temporary, indigestion is uncomfortable.

HAVE A CUP OF CHAMOMILE

Chamomile tea acts as a mild sedative that calms overactive stomach nerves, as well as an antispasmodic that helps to relieve the feelings of cramping that come with indigestion. Simply brew a strong cup of chamomile tea with two teabags, allowing them to steep for at least ten minutes. Drink the tea rapidly as soon as it is cool enough to go down easily.

STIMULATE DIGESTION WITH APPLE CIDER VINEGAR

If you have overeaten, stimulate your digestive tract by drinking a four-ounce glass of water with a teaspoon of apple cider vinegar mixed in. This will increase your stomach's hydrochloric acid production and help alleviate uncomfortable feelings of bloating.

BURP WITH BAKING SODA

To soothe an upset stomach, stir one teaspoon of baking soda into eight ounces of water and drink it slowly. This remedy neutralizes the excess acid in your stomach, turning it into gas and salt. Your body will absorb the salt, and the gas will cause you to burp, relieving the pressure in your stomach.

Ingrown Toenail

A painful ingrown toenail occurs when the corner of one of your toenails grows into the surrounding skin, leading to redness, swelling, and in the worst cases, infection. If you have a severely ingrown toenail that begins to ooze pus, you will not be able to treat it on your own. See a doctor before it gets worse.

LET IT GROW WITH MENTHOL RUB

People often cut their ingrown toenails off, stopping the pain. Unfortunately, this can make the problem worse once the nail grows out again. Ease the pain and allow the toenail to grow out by putting menthol rub on the affected area and covering it with a bandage. The menthol rub will soften the skin and allow the toenail to grow out properly, and the menthol it contains will ease the discomfort. If your toe does not improve within three to four days, seek medical attention.

LIFT IT UP WITH DENTAL FLOSS AND EPSOM SALT

Soak your foot in a basin of hot water with a handful of Epsom salt, allowing it to remain there for ten minutes to soften the skin surrounding your ingrown toenail. Dry your foot and put a triple antibiotic ointment on the affected toe. Next, use a long piece of dental floss to gently lift the corner of the nail from the skin. Trim the ends of the dental floss so that an inch or so protrudes from each side of the nail and leave it in place. Put on comfortable socks. If you need to put on shoes, choose a pair with plenty of toe room. Repeat this treatment, replacing the dental floss daily, for three to four days. If your condition worsens instead of improving, seek medical attention.

PREVENT THE NEXT ONE

The best way to treat an ingrown toenail is not to get one at all, and the methods for avoiding them are surprisingly simple. Most of us round off the corners of our toenails the way we do our fingernails, but this is actually the wrong strategy for toenails. Cut them straight across, allowing the end of the toenail to grow to the tip of the toe. If the sides are too sharp, file them off a little, but allow them to remain square. This is the natural way for the nail to grow, and it will be less likely to round over and grow into your skin. Check your shoe size, too. Be sure your toes have enough room in your shoes. Scrunching your toes in ill-fitting shoes is a sure-fire way to get ingrown nails.

Insect Bites and Stings

Insect bites are often painful and itchy. This happens because insects release chemicals when they bite that trigger minor skin irritation. Bee stings are usually much more painful than bites from other insects, because bees often inject more venom than other species and a bee's stinger creates a larger wound. When you are bitten or stung, resist the urge to scratch at the surrounding tissues, as this will only cause the venom to spread.

REMOVE AN EMBEDDED STINGER WITH A CREDIT CARD

When a bee stings, she dies and leaves her stinger and venom sac behind. Squeezing the stinger in an attempt to remove it can release venom remaining in the sac and make the problem worse. Position the edge of a credit card in front of the venom sac and push down and backward to slide the stinger and sac out in the opposite direction from which they entered your skin. After they have been removed, use one of the following methods to stop the pain.

STOP THE BURNING WITH BAKING SODA

Because baking soda has an alkalizing effect, it neutralizes insect venom, including venom from wasps, bees, and fire ants. Mix a tablespoon of baking soda with about a teaspoon of water to form a thick paste; then cover the affected area.

TRY AN ASPIRIN PASTE

Aspirin contains salicylic acid, which anesthetizes the pain and itching insect bites cause, and which neutralizes insect venom. Smash an aspirin tablet and add a few drops of water to form a thick paste; then apply it to the sting or bite.

DAB ON MENTHOL RUB, PINK BISMUTH, OR TOOTHPASTE

If you have been attacked by mosquitoes, gnats, or chiggers, cover your bites with any of these home remedies and allow it to remain there. Reapply if itching returns. They all contain substances that will soothe the irritation and help keep you from scratching.

Insomnia

Insomnia is the inability to sleep, even when you are exhausted. Stress and caffeine can contribute to the problem, as can watching television and using electronic devices right before bed.

TAKE A LAVENDER BATH

Winding down and allowing your body to relax at bedtime is often just as effective as sleep aids. Draw a hot bath and add two or three drops of lavender essential oil. Relax in the bath for at least fifteen minutes, allowing your thoughts to drift away and focusing on the fragrance of the lavender. Once out of the bathtub, towel off and apply soothing lotion. Put on cozy pajamas and socks, and then lie down in your bed. Close your eyes and drift off to sleep. A lavender bath may be ill-advised for pregnant women as lavender may mimic estrogen. Taking a warm bath without the essential oil—and with the lights turned down low—will also be very relaxing.

PUT THINGS IN PERSPECTIVE

Busy thoughts can keep people from falling asleep, and sleepiness the following day just makes matters worse. If your thoughts often intrude and prevent you from falling asleep when you want to, put things in perspective. About two hours before bedtime, make a list of all the things that are bothering you and allow yourself ten to fifteen minutes to reflect on them and put them into their proper place within the big picture that is life. This will clear your mind. Go for a short walk, read a book, and take a bath or shower, focusing on positive thoughts. Allow yourself to relax completely before settling down for the night.

SIP CHERRY JUICE

Tart cherries and tart cherry juice increase the body's supply of melatonin, which contributes to healthful sleep cycles. Several studies have shown that when consumed regularly, tart cherries work just as well as or better than melatonin supplements and other sleep aids. Drink an eight-ounce glass of tart cherry juice each morning and have another one in the evening. It can take up to two weeks for this remedy to resolve sleep problems completely, but you should notice an improvement within a few days. Keep drinking cherry juice to prevent insomnia from recurring.

INHALE SOME SANDALWOOD ESSENTIAL OIL

Inhale it directly, apply it to your pulse points, or diffuse it in your home or office. You can also add a few drops to a warm bath and relax as you inhale its soothing vapors. (Don't do this if you're pregnant or breast feeding, as there have been reports of miscarriages in women who use sandalwood over the course of several weeks.).

When to See a Doctor A lengthy period of insomnia may indicate a medical issue. It can also cause memory loss, reduced cognitive functioning, and hallucinations. Depression, mini-strokes (also known as transient ischemic attacks or TIAs), and other illnesses can have insomnia as a component. If insomnia lasts more than a few consecutive nights, call your doctor.

Irritable Bowel Syndrome

Irritable bowel syndrome (IBS) is a chronic disorder that affects the way the large intestine works, causing food to move through it either too slowly or too quickly. Symptoms include painful bloating, gas, and abdominal cramps. Dietary modification is the best treatment for IBS, and stress-reduction techniques can also be helpful. Knowing which foods and circumstances tend to bring on symptoms and avoiding those things, if possible, are two important steps to controlling IBS.

SOOTHE SPASMS WITH MINT

Peppermint contains powerful compounds that can often help to ease the spasms that cause IBS-related pain. Drink a cup of hot peppermint tea before and after each meal, and have another one before you go to bed. Avoid artificial sweeteners, as these can sometimes increase IBS symptoms; if you like your tea sweet, use honey.

EASE DISCOMFORT WITH GINGER

Compounds in ginger help suppress prostaglandins, which are substances that control smooth muscle contractions, including those that can bring on intestinal cramping and contractions. The shogaol and gingerol in ginger also help those smooth muscles relax, alleviating painful IBS symptoms. The easiest way to deliver a steady stream of soothing compounds is to drink between four and six cups of ginger tea each day.

KILL IT WITH COCONUT

Coconut and coconut oil have long been known to relieve inflammation in the bowel. Coconut contains a high level of medium-chain triglycerides, a saturated fat that works differently from other fats in the body. While research on coconut is preliminary, some studies report that it can eliminate the bad bacteria in the bowel that causes irritation and unpredictable activity. A tablespoon of coconut a day may make a difference—though many people recommend two or three macaroons daily.

Kidney Stones

Kidney stones are hard masses of salt and minerals found in the urine. They can be as small as a grain of sand or much larger. They form when your body's balance of water, salts, minerals, and other components of urine change. Small stones often pass on their own, but these remedies can help.

DISSOLVE THEM WITH APPLE CIDER VINEGAR

Mild cases of kidney stones often respond well to treatment with organic apple cider vinegar that contains a cloudy substance known as "mother of vinegar." This type of vinegar can be found at most health food stores. Mix two teaspoons of organic apple cider vinegar with eight ounces of water and drink one glass hourly for a twelve-hour period to dissolve stones. Continue drinking the apple cider vinegar and water twice a day to prevent new stones from forming. If you really can't bear the taste of this remedy, add one to two teaspoons of raw honey.

Why It Works Apple cider vinegar contains acetic acid. It may seem counterintuitive that an acid can dissolve crystals that were formed by acid, but vinegar that contains the "mother of vinegar" actually makes urine more alkaline, creating an environment that will dissolve the stones.

DRINK WATER

The most common cause of kidney stones is not drinking enough water. If you tend to get kidney stones, try to drink eight to ten glasses of water a day, so your urine is light yellow.

LEMONADE

Increasing the levels of citrate in the body can help prevent the recurrence of kidney stones. Lemon juice is a good source of this mineral, as is cranberry juice—two drinks that, for most people, taste a lot better than cider vinegar. These beverages also reduce oxalate in the body, a risk factor in the formation of kidney stones.

Macular Degeneration

Can there really be a natural or home remedy that can curb age-related macular degeneration, one of the leading causes of blindness in the elderly? The science is still in progress, but some remedies seem to have an impact on the deterioration of the retina that typifies this condition. The retina works to focus our vision—so if you can't focus, you can't read or do any other kind of close-up work, and that includes using a computer or a smartphone.

LUTEIN AND ZEAXANTHIN

Two carotene compounds found in egg yolks and many green and yellow vegetables may have significant roles to play in reducing macular degeneration. Research conducted at Tufts University has revealed that people who eat a lot of these foods, as well as omega-3 fatty acids, can significantly reduce the risk of developing macular degeneration.

BILBERRY FOR SIGHT

Anecdotal evidence suggests that bilberry, an herb available in nutritional supplement stores, may be good for your eyes. Research has not specifically tested bilberry for its effect on macular degeneration, but it has shown that the herb may reduce overgrowth of blood vessels, a symptom of macular degeneration. As bilberry is not known for interactions with prescription medications, trying out this herbal supplement is unlikely to have any serious side effects.

PRESERVE EYESIGHT WITH FISH

Eating fatty fishes that contain omega-3 fatty acids can leave you less likely to develop macular degeneration. In addition, the Age-Related Eye Disease Study determined that vitamins C and E, beta carotene, and zinc and copper work together to prevent age-related eye diseases.

Menopause Symptoms

Women sometimes experience uncomfortable symptoms as they enter menopause. These include hot flashes, interrupted sleep, and emotional turbulence, and are caused by a drop in natural progesterone and estrogen levels.

DRINK SOY MILK

Adding soy to your diet is an excellent way to alleviate the uncomfortable symptoms that accompany menopause, because soy can increase estrogen levels. To feel more like yourself again, consume thirty-two ounces of soy milk daily. Use it to replace dairy products you may add to beverages such as coffee and tea, have some on your cereal, and enjoy creamy fruit smoothies. You'll find that this strategy makes it easy to consume enough soy to make a difference.

TAKE VITAMIN B₆

Take 100 mg of vitamin B_6 each day to alleviate menopausal mood swings. If supplements aren't for you, increase your intake of leafy green vegetables, avocados, and asparagus, all of which are good sources of the vitamin.

Why It Works Vitamin B_6 is required for the production of serotonin, a neurotransmitter than helps control mood swings and other mental and emotional symptoms of menopause. Boosting your B_6 levels can help stabilize your moods, helping you avoid depression as well as erratic changes in temperament.

WALK FOR THIRTY MINUTES

Walking for as little as thirty minutes each day helps reduce menopausal symptoms of anxiety, stress, and depression. Also, hormonal changes increase your risk of heart disease and cause weight gain, making exercise an ally in protecting your health.

Menstrual Cramps

Menstrual cramps may result when the uterus contracts to expel the unneeded uterine lining built up during the previous month. In severe cases, you may need to take a pain reliever such as naproxen or ibuprofen, but home remedies often work just as well.

DRINK GINGER TEA

Ginger contains compounds that suppress prostaglandins, which are responsible for the uterine contractions that trigger cramping. It also contains shogaol and gingerol, which help the muscles relax. Brew a strong cup of ginger tea with two teabags that contain real ginger. Inhale the vapors as it cools, and drink it plain or with a little honey. Repeat this treatment three times a day during your period to keep cramping at a minimum.

APPLY CLARY SAGE ESSENTIAL OIL

To alleviate menstrual cramps and premenstrual symptoms, apply diluted clary sage essential oil to your pulse points and temples. Blend a drop or two into a cup of warm water or hot herbal tea and enjoy. You can also diffuse it in your home or office and inhale it directly.

Why It Works Clary sage oil contains the anti-inflammatory compounds linalyl acetate and myrcene, which may assist in dismissing the pain of menstrual cramps.

BOOST CIRCULATION WITH EXERCISE

Moderate exercise boosts circulation, which in turn diminishes cramping. Just twenty minutes of walking, cycling, swimming, or playing a sport you enjoy will also give your mood a boost and soothe stress by increasing endorphin levels.

Migraine

Migraines are recurring headaches that can range from mild to debilitating, and that can last as long as seventy-two hours. A number of factors trigger migraines; sometimes they occur with hormonal changes, and in some cases they are triggered by certain foods such as chocolate or aged cheese. To treat a migraine, place a damp cloth on your head, close your eyes, and stay away from bright lights. If migraines happen frequently or if you suffer from a severe, sudden migraine that is accompanied by blurred vision, you should seek medical attention.

CHANGE YOUR DIET

A remarkable number of foods and beverages have emerged as migraine triggers. The most pernicious are the ones that contain tyramine or phenylethylamine, the amino acids found in aged or fermented cheeses, soy foods, nuts, citrus fruits, and red wine and balsamic vinegar. In addition, migraines have been linked directly to tannins in red wine and red fruits, and to chocolate, alcoholic beverages, and chemical additives in processed foods: nitrates, sulfites, monosodium glutamate, and aspartame. There is no easy way to determine which of these foods and additives may be triggering your own migraines. Doctors and purveyors of alternative therapies generally recommend that you strip down your diet to a fairly restricted assortment of foods that are not known migraine triggers, then add in other foods gradually to determine which ones might be causing your debilitating headaches. If you suffer from particularly miserable migraines, you may be willing to go through this time-consuming process in the hope that you will never have another one.

DRINK TEA

Although caffeine can help alleviate migraine pain by constricting swollen blood vessels, coffee contains compounds that can cause some migraines to worsen. Black or orange pekoe tea contains enough caffeine to make a difference, but it lacks the chemicals that make migraines worse. Sweeten your tea with honey rather than sugar or artificial sweetener.

BATHE IN PEPPERMINT ESSENTIAL OIL

Peppermint essential oil addresses migraine symptoms in multiple ways, cooling and relaxing muscles and blood vessels, stimulating the nervous system, and soothing the nausea that sometimes comes with a severe migraine. Simply fill your bathtub with hot water and add five drops of peppermint essential oil. Relax as you inhale the vapors, remaining in the bath for at least fifteen minutes. After toweling off and dressing, prepare a cup of peppermint tea made with eight ounces of hot water and one or two drops of peppermint essential oil.

Morning Sickness

Despite its name, the nausea and vomiting associated with morning sickness can happen at any time of the day or night during pregnancy. Morning sickness is most prevalent during the first trimester but sometimes lasts longer.

HAVE SALTINES AND GINGER ALE

The sugar and ginger in ginger ale help to alleviate the nausea associated with morning sickness. Be sure to choose ginger ale that contains real ginger. Several natural brands are available. If the gassiness of soda bothers you, let the ginger ale go flat by leaving the cap off the bottle. Meanwhile, saltine crackers are bland and have a lot of starch. This high level of starch helps absorb excess stomach acid and relieves nausea.

DRINK WATER AND SNACK FREQUENTLY

One of the easiest ways to prevent morning sickness is to stay hydrated by drinking one eight-ounce glass of water during each hour you are awake. This helps to keep stomach acid from building up. Snacking at regular intervals helps as well, keeping your blood sugar levels constant.

ENJOY HERBAL TEA

Herbal teas made with ginger, lemon balm, or peppermint are excellent for reducing nausea. If one of your morning sickness symptoms is heartburn, stick to ginger or lemon balm tea, since heartburn often worsens with peppermint.

TAKE VITAMIN B_6

Studies show that vitamin B_6 aids in alleviating the nausea and vomiting that make morning sickness so miserable. Women who participated in the studies took 25 mg of the vitamin three times a day and experienced relief after an average of three days. Be sure to talk with your doctor before including vitamin B_6 in your daily regimen.

LOVE YOURSELF WITH LEMON

Most people enjoy the fragrance of fresh lemon, and many enjoy its flavor as well. The aroma and taste of lemon triggers the digestive system to speed up. This eases nausea and helps reduce the urge to vomit. Some women find that just smelling fresh lemon alleviates symptoms, while others find it best to eat a slice of lemon or drink a tablespoon of fresh lemon juice. The fragrance and flavor of other citrus fruits sometimes helps, too; try tangerines, oranges, or clementines.

Motion Sickness

Motion sickness occurs when the parts of the body that detect motion, such as the inner ear and the eyes, send unexpected or conflicting messages to the brain. This happens in the presence of unsteady movement, such as a car on a bumpy road or a ship riding over the waves. It can also happen when what you see is out of synch with what your body is experiencing, such as while playing an intense video game with simulated motion. The conflict between the senses results in motion sickness.

STICK TO LOW-FAT FOODS

If you're going to ride in a car, fly in a plane, or spend time on a boat, stay away from greasy foods or dishes that are hard to digest. But don't skip a meal—that can be even worse for developing queasiness by disrupting the electrical signals between your eyes, ears, and stomach. Choose fruits, vegetables, and whole grains over a cheeseburger and fries.

BRING THE ACUPRESSURE BANDS

Sea-Bands, a common product in airport newsstands and other travel stores, are elastic bands you wear around both wrists. Each band has a plastic knob that presses gently against a specific point on your wrist. The result is a signal to your brain to hold steady. It may seem like new-age hocus-pocus, but many people can tell you from experience that this works—and it beats taking medications that makes you too drowsy to enjoy the trip.

ENJOY GINGER CANDY

Natural ginger candy is an excellent remedy for motion sickness, because it neutralizes indigestion and helps prevent the brain from signaling the body to vomit defensively. Have a ginger candy or a piece of candied ginger an hour before you begin to travel, and keep eating it throughout your trip, enjoying a piece every half hour or so. Be sure to choose a brand that contains natural ginger rather than artificial flavors.

WATCH THE HORIZON

Stop motion sickness by minimizing the sensory input that causes it. You can do this by watching the horizon or fixing your gaze on a stable point in front of you. If you are a passenger in a train or car, try to sit in the car's front seat or near the front of the train compartment, so you can see where you are going. If you cannot do this, close your eyes, lean back, and try to go to sleep.

Mouth Burns

Almost everyone has suffered a burned mouth or tongue after biting into food that's too hot or sipping a scalding beverage. When left untreated, these burned spots can take up to a week to heal on their own.

SUCK ON AN ICE CUBE

One of the fastest ways to stop a burned mouth from hurting and to promote healing is to suck on an ice cube. Pop the ice cube in your mouth, using your tongue to press it against the burned area. Keep sucking on the ice cube until it melts. If you like, you can enjoy a popsicle or another frozen treat instead.

SWISH PINK BISMUTH

Ease the pain and swelling caused by a mouth burn with a tablespoon of pink bismuth. Swish it around in your mouth, coating the affected area. Hold your tongue still and try not to speak or swallow for at least five minutes, so the remedy has a chance to work. Milk is effective as a soothing coating as well.

VITAMIN E FOR BURNS

Pierce and squeeze a 1,000 mg vitamin E capsule over the burned area. This can be tricky if the burn is on your tongue, especially if you don't like the taste, but if you've burned a cheek or other areas in your mouth, you may find this remedy particularly effective. Vitamin E helps heal burned skin and regenerate healthy skin cells, speeding healing to your mouth.

Muscle Cramps

Cramps are caused by muscle spasms, during which muscles contract involuntarily. These spasms usually affect muscles located in the feet, calves, and thighs, although they can also affect muscles in the abdomen, the back, the ribcage, and the hands and arms. Cramps can occur because of muscle fatigue but are often triggered by depleted sodium, potassium, and electrolyte levels.

STRETCH IT OUT IMMEDIATELY

The pain of a leg or foot cramp can be sharp and severe enough to cause you to panic. The best thing to do is stretch that muscle to release the cramping. If the cramp is in your foot, stand up and flex your toes, applying pressure in the opposite direction of the cramp to release it. If it's in your lower leg, flexing your foot in one direction or the other may provide the motion your muscle needs to relax.

HAVE A SPORTS DRINK

Sports drinks such as Gatorade contain sodium, potassium, and electrolytes. They are formulated to deliver these nutrients to the body's tissues quickly, and can help alleviate cramping.

INCREASE CALCIUM AND POTASSIUM

Adding more skim milk, cheese, and yogurt to your diet can increase your intake of calcium, something your muscles need to function properly. Potatoes and bananas are good sources of potassium, a mineral that most Americans need to increase in their diet. Both of these minerals can help reduce leg cramps.

ENJOY A SOAK WITH EPSOM SALT

Warming muscles quickly relieves cramping in most cases. The easiest way to warm large muscle groups is to take a hot bath, preferably with two cups of Epsom salt added to the water. The magnesium in Epsom salt helps muscles relax more quickly than hot water alone.

Nail Fungus

If your fingernails and toenails are thick and brown or yellow, you have a nail fungus. For many people, this requires no treatment—it's more of a cosmetic nuisance than a true medical issue. If you are diabetic, however, any kind of infection poses a health risk.

SOAK IT IN VINEGAR

Mix equal parts of vinegar and warm water together in a basin. If the fungus is on your toenails, soak your feet in the vinegar bath for fifteen to thirty minutes. If your fingernails are affected, soak your hands in the basin. Dry the nails thoroughly afterward. Do this twice daily until the discoloration disappears and your nails return to normal.

TEA TREE OIL

Dab a little tea tree oil on your affected fingernails and toenails. Repeat this several times a day until the discoloration disappears.

Why It Works Tea tree oil has natural antiseptic properties that make it particularly effective in killing fungus. Small studies have shown promising results in using tea tree oil to kill fungi, yeast infections (athlete's foot), and other skin conditions. It should not be taken internally.

SOAK IN CORNMEAL MUSH

Farmers have used cornmeal mush on their crops for centuries to kill fungus in the ground around the plants. Remarkably, it works for fingernail and toenail fungus, as well. Here's how to use it.

1. Get a basin large enough to soak your feet in. Spread cornmeal in the bottom of the basin, about 1 inch thick.
2. Pour in 10 cups of room-temperature water. Don't mix it up! Let the ingredients sit for 1 hour, so the water and cornmeal combine on their own.
3. Add more water until there's about an inch of water over the mush.
4. Soak your foot (or feet) for 30 minutes. Make sure that the water and mush cover your whole foot, so you kill the fungus spores beyond your toenails.
5. Rinse your feet and pat them dry.
6. Do all of this twice a day until your toenails return to their normal color.

Nausea

Feelings of queasiness and the urge to vomit accompany nausea. There are many reasons you might feel nauseous, including motion sickness, a stomach virus, exposure to a foul odor, indigestion, or a bad headache.

TRY PEPPERMINT TEA

One of the best remedies for nausea is natural peppermint tea made with dried peppermint leaves. This contains just enough menthol to calm the stomach's lining and stop feelings of queasiness. Brew a cup of tea using one teabag and eight ounces of hot water, adding honey to sweeten it if you like. Inhale the vapors as it cools.

EAT GINGERSNAPS

Natural ginger contains compounds that soothe the stomach and stop spasms associated with nausea. Gingersnaps made with natural ginger also contain carbohydrates, which can help settle the stomach. Have three gingersnaps and a cup of hot tea, preferably made with ginger or peppermint teabags, relaxing and breathing deeply as you enjoy your snack. If you still feel nauseous, lie down for fifteen minutes or try to take a longer nap if you have time.

INHALE GINGER ESSENTIAL OIL

You may inhale ginger essential oil after diluting it with carrier oil. Apply a few drops to a cloth and inhale deeply. This is an excellent way to deal with nausea.

Nosebleed

Nosebleeds can be caused by trauma or by irritated nasal linings caused by flu, cold, or even dry heat. Allergies, high blood pressure, and damage caused by nose picking can also lead to nosebleeds.

COAT THE NASAL PASSAGES WITH WITCH HAZEL

Witch hazel contains astringents that help constrict blood vessels and stop nosebleeds. Use it to soak a cotton swab, and then gently apply the liquid to the inside of the affected nostril. While you are waiting for the astringent to take effect, hold your head level and breathe through your mouth as you gently pinch the fleshy portion of your nose.

TRY WHITE VINEGAR

If you have white vinegar available, it can help seal the blood vessel wall. Soak a cloth or cotton ball with vinegar and place it in the nostril that is bleeding. Leave it in place for ten minutes, keeping your head level and breathing through your mouth so you don't inadvertently swallow blood.

GRAB A BAG OF PEAS

Pressing a bag of frozen vegetables—or a plastic bag filled with ice, if you don't have veggies on hand—against the bridge of your nose will constrict the blood vessels and slow down the bleeding. Keep the icy compress in place until the bleeding stops.

Painful Gums

Minor gum pain is usually an indicator that you should brush and floss your teeth better or more often. If you have a serious case of gingivitis with red, swollen gums, you could be in danger of losing your teeth. Be sure to make an appointment with your dentist to have potentially serious problems addressed before that happens.

RINSE WITH HYDROGEN PEROXIDE

Hydrogen peroxide kills bacteria that contribute to gum pain while simultaneously relieving soreness. Make a rinse by blending one tablespoon of hydrogen peroxide with one tablespoon of warm water, and use it to rinse your mouth for at least thirty seconds. Do not swallow. Repeat as needed.

SEA SALT SOLUTION

Sea salt not only reduces the swelling in your gums but it also has the ability to draw bacteria and infection out of any abscesses. A sea salt solution can help relieve the worst of the pain until you can get in to see your dentist. Dissolve a teaspoon of sea salt in a cup of warm water, and swish it in your mouth for thirty seconds. Spit it out and do it again three or four times. Once you've alleviated the initial pain, continue to use this mouth rinse twice a day after you brush your teeth to help you avoid any recurrence.

Why It Works Sea salt has magnesium, potassium, calcium, and other minerals that provide healing elements, promote saliva production (which protects teeth), and protect the teeth from acidic damage. These minerals and trace elements have been removed from processed table salt, though both salts contain similar amounts of sodium.

APPLY ALOE VERA GEL

Aloe vera gel soothes gum irritation and stimulates circulation, encouraging damaged gums to heal. Apply a thin coating of gel with a cotton swab or a soft-bristled toothbrush. Try not to swallow for at least ten minutes so the gel has the opportunity to work.

Poison Ivy

Poison ivy, poison oak, and poison sumac all contain an irritant called urushiol, which is an oily, sticky substance that adheres to your skin. If you come into contact with any of these plants, washing your skin within fifteen minutes can help to prevent the painful, itchy rash that typically develops following exposure. Be sure to remove clothes that have come into contact with the plants, as well, and launder them in hot soapy water as soon as possible. Urushiol contaminates everything it touches, so the inside of your car, your furniture, and even your pets can be affected.

USE BABY WIPES

If you're spending time in an area where poison ivy or its relatives are present, keep baby wipes with you. Use them to wash areas immediately when you suspect exposure. The alcohol in the baby wipes cuts through the oily urushiol and can save you from developing a rash and blisters. Try to shower within one hour to further reduce the risk of a rash.

BATHE IN INSTANT ICED TEA

Instant iced tea powder contains high levels of tannin, which calms itching, helps dry blisters, and soothes irritated skin. If you have developed a poison ivy rash, draw a warm bath and add a cup of instant iced tea powder to it. Spend at least fifteen minutes in the bathtub.

ENJOY AN OATMEAL SOAK

Oats have anti-inflammatory properties that help soothe the itching, burning discomfort caused by exposure to poison ivy and related plants. To make an extra-strength oatmeal bath, put two cups of rolled oats in the blender or food processer and pulse to chop them coarsely. Use a funnel to pour the chopped oats into an old dress sock or one leg of a pair of used pantyhose, and tie a knot to keep the oats from escaping. Run a warm bath, positioning the oats beneath the faucet. Leave the oats in the water while you soak. Spend at least fifteen minutes in the bathtub.

Premenstrual Syndrome (PMS)

Premenstrual syndrome (PMS) causes symptoms that include fatigue, irritability, food cravings, and mood swings; all can begin as early as two weeks before your monthly cycle. Poor eating habits, stress, and hormonal fluctuations can make symptoms worse.

HAVE A HIGH-FIBER BREAKFAST

Eating plenty of fiber at breakfast helps keep estrogen levels stable and prevent wild mood swings. Choose fruit, bran flakes, oatmeal, and other foods that contain fiber. Aim for at least 20 g of fiber at breakfast and try to get another 15 to 20 g of fiber throughout the rest of the day.

REACH FOR ROSEMARY ESSENTIAL OIL

Compounds in rosemary essential oil help alleviate PMS symptoms by stabilizing hormone levels. Keep a bottle of pure rosemary essential oil near you. When you start to feel irritable, tired, or hungry for unhealthful food, sprinkle a drop or two on a soft cloth, inhaling deeply. You can also dab a drop of rosemary essential oil behind each ear to maximize its effects, as long as you do not have sensitive skin.

Why It Works Rosemary has been shown in clinical studies to be an effective remedy for reducing anxiety and stress, and for the alteration of pain perception. This may be why rosemary has been used to treat painful menstruation for centuries.

TRY CLARY SAGE ESSENTIAL OIL

To alleviate menstrual cramps and premenstrual symptoms, apply diluted clary sage essential oil to your pulse points and temples. Blend a drop or two into a cup of warm water or hot herbal tea and enjoy. You can also diffuse it in your home or office and inhale it directly.

Receding Gums

Healthy teeth and gums are important to your overall health. Be sure to brush and floss your teeth, and consider using mouthwash to help keep the bacteria that contribute to dental problems at bay.

HEAL WITH TEA TREE OIL

Receding gums are usually caused by a chronic minor bacterial infection, and while brushing and flossing carefully after each meal will work wonders to bring your gums back to health, you can help them heal faster with tea tree essential oil. Just place several drops on your toothbrush after each brushing and apply it to your teeth and gums. You can soak dental floss in tea tree oil to get into the tight spaces your toothbrush can't reach. Continue using this remedy until your gums return to health.

RINSE WITH SEA SALT

Long recommended by dentists, sea salt provides fluoride and minerals such as calcium and magnesium, helping you keep your teeth and gums healthy. While studies have not yet been conducted to prove sea salt's ability to draw out infection from abscesses, dentists can supply plenty of anecdotal evidence to support this practice.

BLEND SEA SALT AND BAKING SODA

If the sea salt rinse did you some good, try this homemade tooth powder:

1. Blend together 6 parts baking soda with 1 part sea salt, using your food processor for 30 seconds, or mixing the ingredients in a cup by hand.
2. Wet your index finger and dip it into the cup of baking soda and salt.
3. Rub the soda and salt mixture gently on your gums, starting on the outside and working your way around. Re-dip your finger in the powder as necessary.
4. When all your teeth and gums have been coated, wait 5 minutes, then rinse your mouth with water and spit out the remaining powder.

Restless Legs Syndrome

Restless legs syndrome (RLS) includes symptoms such as itchy, tickling, aching legs, along with muscle spasms in the legs. The irresistible desire to move the legs is also a hallmark of RLS. There are many causes of restless legs syndrome, including iron deficiency, varicose veins, fibromyalgia, and diabetes. If you suffer from RLS and home remedies do not stop your symptoms, see a doctor immediately to rule out a serious underlying condition.

EXERCISE AND STRETCH REGULARLY

The muscles, blood vessels, and arteries in your legs and feet need to move to function properly. If you have a sedentary job or have a tendency to spend your spare time surfing the Internet or watching television, lack of exercise is probably one of the main contributors to your RLS problem. The best remedy is regular exercise; just walking for twenty to thirty minutes each day is usually enough to stop the spasms. Stretch your legs after you have walked five minutes and stretch again after you finish walking. Stretching before bed can also be helpful.

CORRECT THE IRON DEFICIENCY

According to Johns Hopkins, "The single most consistent finding and the strongest environmental risk factor associated with RLS is iron insufficiency," so increasing the iron in your diet can go a long way in relieving your symptoms. In particular, clams, oysters, organ meats, beef, pork, poultry, and fish are recommended for increasing your iron intake. If you are a vegetarian or if you have other reasons for avoiding these foods, taking a daily iron supplement may bring you relief from the sensations.

TAKE A LAVENDER BATH

If symptoms wake you up at night and will not stop, soothe your legs by taking a hot bath with a few drops of lavender essential oil added to the water to help your mind and body relax. Remain in the bathtub for at least fifteen minutes, stretching the muscles in your legs to help relieve cramping.

Ringworm

Despite its name, ringworm is caused by a fungus, not parasites. It is characterized by raised, circular patches and severe itchiness. Ringworm is extremely contagious and is passed to others by contact. It is often contracted in public restrooms and other venues where people tend to congregate. If you have ringworm, do not scratch yourself, as this is the fastest way to spread the fungus on your own body, and to transfer it on your hands to others. If home remedies do not provide relief or help your ringworm heal, seek medical attention.

DAB ON MYRRH ESSENTIAL OIL

Myrrh essential oil is a strong antifungal agent that can kill ringworm. Using a cotton swab, apply a light coat directly to the affected area three to four times a day, discarding the swab immediately after use. Patches of ringworm should start to disappear after about a week, and should be completely clear within three weeks.

EAT AND APPLY GARLIC

Garlic helps the body fight fungal infections from the inside out. While you use a topical remedy to soothe the itch, increase your garlic intake significantly to boost your ability to fight off the ringworm infection. You can also use fresh garlic to create a topical treatment for ringworm. Place two peeled cloves of garlic in the blender with ½ teaspoon of water. Scoop out the resulting paste and apply it to affected areas as needed, using a cotton swab to prevent contamination and discarding it after use. Leave the garlic in place until it has dried; then wash it away.

USE TEA TREE ESSENTIAL OIL

Tea tree essential oil is a powerful antifungal agent. Using a cotton swab, dab a light coat onto the affected area three to four times daily, discarding the swab after use. Patches of ringworm should lighten within a week, and should be clear within three weeks.

Scrapes

A scrape is an injury that tears away part of the upper layer of skin. Painful and sometimes filled with debris, scrapes need to be cleaned before they can be effectively treated. If you have a deep scrape with debris you are unable to remove on your own, seek medical treatment to prevent a serious infection.

LIFT DEBRIS WITH HYDROGEN PEROXIDE

Hydrogen peroxide's bubbling action can help lift lightweight debris, such as grass and other plant matter, from a scrape. Allow the scrape to bleed freely for up to a minute, as this is the body's method of pushing debris out. Next, pour a liberal amount of hydrogen peroxide onto the scrape, allowing debris and excess liquid to flow off. Rinse the wound with water and then apply a triple antibiotic ointment and cover it with a bandage. Reapply the ointment and change the bandage at least once a day, watching for signs of infection, including swelling and redness. If you see these signs, get medical treatment.

APPLY LAVENDER OIL

Lavender essential oil has antibacterial and antiseptic properties that make it particularly effective in healing scrapes. It's also soothing, which provides the added benefit of reducing pain and inflammation. Put two or three drops on a cotton ball or pad and apply it to the scrape. Cover the scrape with a gauze pad or adhesive bandage, and change the bandage daily until the scrape heals.

HEAL WITH HONEY

If you have a small scrape, you can use honey to help it heal faster. Wash the scrape with soap and water right after it happens. Coat it with a thin layer of honey and cover it with a bandage. Reapply the honey and change the bandage daily until the scrape heals.

Seasonal Allergies

Seasonal allergies caused by exposure to certain pollens or spores that the body interprets as harmful substances can lead to sneezing, watery eyes, a runny nose, and sinus pressure. Some seasonal allergy symptoms are so severe that they require medical intervention. If home remedies and nonprescription allergy medication don't work for you, see your doctor for a stronger solution.

TAKE A DETOXIFYING BATH

Detoxification enables your body to deal with allergens and helps convince it to release histamines all at once. After you take a detoxifying bath, your body requires several hours to build up its histamine load again, giving you relief from symptoms during that time. Draw a hot bath and immerse your entire body in it for five minutes. Drain the bathtub and take a hot shower, staying in the shower for ten minutes. Towel off and dress comfortably.

KEEP POLLEN OUTDOORS

Minimize your symptoms by keeping pollen outdoors. Keep windows and doors closed during allergy season. Change your clothes as soon as you come in from outside, placing them in a tightly closed laundry hamper. Have other family members do the same, and make sure everyone removes their shoes before walking through the house. Use high-efficiency particulate absorption (HEPA) filters to capture any stray pollen particles that make their way into your living space. When you do go out, wear a paper surgical mask over your mouth and nose to minimize how much pollen you breathe in.

DRINK BLACK TEA WITH LOCAL HONEY

Black tea contains flavonoids that inhibit inflammation, and it helps thin mucus secretions so stuffiness stays at a minimum. Add two teaspoons of raw honey from a local apiary to your tea to boost your tolerance to plants and flowers that are common in your area. Consume raw local honey all year long to develop greater resistance to allergens.

Sinus Pressure

When sinus linings become inflamed and swollen, the resulting pressure can cause terrible headaches. Normal drainage is impeded and can cause mucus to back up, making the problem worse.

HAVE SOME HORSERADISH

Horseradish is a very spicy condiment that penetrates nasal congestion and opens up sinuses, encouraging them to drain. Have a box of tissues on standby and swallow a teaspoon of horseradish. The pressure should clear up instantly.

TAKE A EUCALYPTUS BATH

Eucalyptus essential oil contains powerful compounds that encourage sinuses to drain rapidly. Fill your bathtub with hot water and add six drops of eucalyptus essential oil. Close the shower curtain to contain the vapors and allow the steam to penetrate your sinuses. Use tissues to blow your nose while relaxing in the bath.

STEAM OPEN SINUSES

Steam dilates the blood vessels in your sinuses and helps open them up. Fill a teacup with boiling water and place your nose and mouth over the opening. Breathe in and relax.

Sore Throat

The burning pain, difficulty swallowing, and internal swelling of a sore throat are usually associated with colds and the flu. While home remedies work most of the time, a sore throat that doesn't respond to treatment within five to seven days could signify a serious underlying condition, such as strep throat. See a doctor if your sore throat gets worse or stays the same, rather than improving.

GARGLE WITH APPLE CIDER VINEGAR

Gargling with apple cider vinegar kills bacteria and helps soothe the pain of a sore throat. Make a solution with one tablespoon of warm water and one tablespoon of apple cider vinegar, and gargle with it hourly while you are awake.

DRINK HONEY AND LEMON

Mix one teaspoon of fresh lemon juice with three teaspoons of honey, and then drink it all at once. Wait at least fifteen minutes before eating or drinking anything else, so the honey and lemon have time to soothe your throat and reduce inflammation.

GARGLE WITH SALT WATER

To relieve a sore throat with salt water, mix ½ teaspoon of salt into eight ounces of lukewarm water, stirring until the salt has dissolved. Use the salt water to gargle for about thirty seconds at a time, continuing the treatment every thirty minutes or so, as needed.

Spider Bites

Spider bites can be swollen, itchy, and very painful, because they carry a lot of venom. Most spider bites are not serious, and home remedies can help soothe the itch and take away the sting. If you have a spider bite that causes extreme swelling and redness, serious burning pain, or difficulty breathing, or if you have been bitten by a poisonous species such as a black widow or brown recluse, seek emergency medical treatment as quickly as possible.

EASE THE BURN WITH ICE

Slow the spread of venom and ease burning around spider bites by applying an ice pack. Elevate the affected area, if possible.

BANISH VENOM WITH BAKING SODA

Baking soda neutralizes venom and stops pain and stinging associated with spider bites. Make a paste with one teaspoon of baking soda and one teaspoon of water and apply it directly to the spider bite. Allow it to dry. Reapply as needed to keep itchiness and stinging at bay.

When to See a Doctor If you have difficulty breathing, nausea, muscle spasms, a tightening in your throat, sweating, and dizziness or feel faint, get to an emergency room immediately. Symptoms of a poisonous spider bite include fever and chills, a whole-body skin rash with tiny purple and red spots, nausea, vomiting, and joint pain. If you are bitten by a black widow or brown recluse spider, go to an emergency room immediately.

Splinter

Splinters or wood slivers cause quite a bit of pain, even though they are often small. Try one of these simple home remedies to make removal easy.

DRAW IT OUT WITH DUCT TAPE

Cut a small piece of duct tape and stick it over the splinter. Pull it off, and a splinter that is not too deep in the skin should come out with it.

EASE IT OUT WITH HYDROGEN PEROXIDE

Hydrogen peroxide can lift a splinter out of the skin. Pour a small amount of hydrogen peroxide into a cup or bowl and soak the affected area in it for three minutes. The peroxide should surround the splinter and carry it out of your skin.

LUBRICATE IT WITH OLIVE OIL

Dab some olive oil onto the splinter and cover the affected area with a bandage. After ten minutes or so, use a pair of tweezers to pull the splinter out. It should slip away easily from your skin.

Sprain

Minor sprains involve muscle pain and swelling in the surrounding area. It's best to have sprains checked by a doctor, but home remedies can help stop the pain and reduce the potential for worse injury in the meantime.

REST AND ELEVATE IT

Stop using the injured limb immediately, since even minor movements can make matters worse. Relax in a comfortable position and elevate the injured body part.

ICE IT

Apply an ice pack to the injury to ease inflammation and help stop any internal bleeding. Use the ice pack for fifteen to twenty minutes at a time, repeating every two to three hours. Be sure to put a towel between your skin and the ice pack to prevent a cold injury to your skin.

COMPRESS IT

Use an elastic bandage to compress the area until it stops swelling. The bandage should not be so tight that it cuts off the circulation, but it should be firm. Watch for swelling below the wrapped area; if this occurs, loosen the wrap.

Sty

A sty is basically a pimple that forms in the upper or lower eyelid. It is an infection, usually caused by a blocked oil duct combined with bacteria that normally live on the surface of the eyelid. A simple sty will often heal on its own, and this remedy will help. While you are treating your sty, do not wear contact lenses or eye makeup. Avoid the urge to squeeze or pop the sty, as this can cause the infection to spread. If the sty does not heal or appears to be getting worse, see your eye doctor.

APPLY HEAT

Use a warm, moist compress to bring relief quickly. Just run hot water over a clean washcloth, wring it out, close your eye, and hold it in place until the washcloth cools. Repeat this several times over the course of about ten to fifteen minutes. Repeat the treatment four times a day for a week, using a clean washcloth for each treatment.

PREVENT THE NEXT ONE

Keep your eyelids and eyelashes clean to prevent the blockage in an oil duct that results in a sty. Remove makeup thoroughly in the evening before bed, and wash away any products, sweat, dirt, or anything else that accumulates around the eye during the course of a day.

ADD OMEGA-3S

Omega-3 fatty acids are associated with keeping ducts and glands clean and functioning properly throughout the body. Increasing foods like salmon, halibut, albacore, trout, herring, shrimp, clams, chunk light tuna, catfish, cod, spinach, walnuts, and flaxseed and canola oil can increase the levels of this polyunsaturated fat in your body.

Sunburn

Sunburn is caused by overexposure to radiation from the sun's ultraviolet rays. The faster you treat a sunburn, the less likely it is to blister and peel. If you suffer from a serious sunburn with deep blisters, you may need professional medical care. Some of the worst cases result in hospitalization. The best way to treat a sunburn is to prevent it by applying sunscreen regularly.

COOL IT WITH ALOE

Aloe vera gel is an excellent remedy for sunburn. When applied immediately, fresh aloe gel promotes rapid healing, cooling the discomfort and hydrating the skin. In some cases, aloe can heal sunburns in a surprisingly short amount of time. Apply it liberally to the affected area and repeat as needed.

EASE PAIN WITH WHITE VINEGAR

Vinegar contains acetic acid, which helps to stop pain and soothe inflammation. Make a solution with four ounces of white vinegar and four ounces of water. Pour it into a clean spray bottle and apply it liberally to affected areas, allowing it to dry naturally. Repeat as necessary.

SOAK IN APPLE CIDER VINEGAR

Add a cup of apple cider vinegar to a lukewarm bath and soak in it for ten minutes to help ease the pain of sunburn.

Swimmer's Ear

Swimmer's ear is caused by moisture trapped in the outer ear, where bacteria are able to proliferate. This causes feelings of discomfort and itchiness that can become worse if the ear is left untreated. If you notice swelling or pain, or if your ear does not improve within three days, be sure to consult your doctor immediately.

KILL BACTERIA WITH WHITE VINEGAR

The acid in white vinegar kills the bacteria that cause swimmer's ear. Lie down on your side, with the affected ear up. Use an eyedropper to fill your ear canal with vinegar. Allow it to remain there for five minutes, then lie on your other side with your affected ear over a towel and allow it to drain. Repeat this treatment twice a day for up to three days.

SOOTHE AND DISINFECT WITH GARLIC OIL

Warm garlic has been associated with ear-pain relief in homeopathic circles for decades, though scientists have not fully explored the reasons for this relationship. Suffice to say that a few drops of warmed garlic oil in the ear canal can ease the pain and appears to kill bacteria in the ear as well. Keep the oil in the ear for about ten minutes, and then allow it to drain onto a cotton ball placed outside the ear.

PREVENT IT WITH MINERAL OIL

Public swimming pools are often a breeding ground for bacteria. To prevent swimmer's ear, place a few drops of mineral oil into each of your ears before you get into the water. This creates a barrier that helps keep water and bacteria away from the skin inside your ears.

Tick Bites

Ticks inhabit low-lying brush, trees, and grass. Their bites can cause irritation and itching. Most tick bites are benign, but some do carry diseases such as Rocky Mountain spotted fever and Lyme disease. If you suspect that you have been exposed to a tick-borne infection, seek medical treatment immediately.

REMOVE THE TICK

As soon as you discover the tick in your skin, carefully remove it. The sooner it's out, the less likely it is that a disease-carrying tick will have the chance to spread its infection.

1. Use tweezers with a fine tip.
2. Grab the tick with the tweezers, getting as close as you can to its mouth. The mouth is the part that's holding onto your skin.
3. Be careful not to grab the tick by its body, as you could end up squeezing infected fluid into your skin.
4. Pull the tick straight out. Do not twist it, or you may break the parasite and cause the fluid to flow.
5. Drop the tick into a resealable plastic bag or an empty jar. You may need it for identification later to determine if it may have given you a disease.
6. Wash the bite with warm, soapy water. Many sources recommend using a dish soap like Dawn or Ivory.
7. Apply an antibiotic ointment to the bite, and cover it with an adhesive bandage.

8. Wash your hands. Wash them again.
9. Examine the rest of your body for more ticks, especially if you've been out hiking in the woods in an area known for having lots of ticks.

APPLY ICE

An ice pack can help reduce the swelling and itching associated with a tick bite. Ice your bite for fifteen to twenty minutes every hour for six hours. Resist the urge to scratch, since this can spread venom.

EASE PAIN WITH ASPIRIN PASTE

Aspirin contains salicylic acid, which neutralizes the venom that causes stinging and itching. Crush an adult aspirin tablet and add a few drops of water to it to form a paste. Apply the paste to the tick bite and leave it there until it dries. Repeat as needed.

When to See a Doctor If you develop chills, fever, headache, joint pain, muscle pain, a stiff neck, or a general feeling of malaise, you may be coming down with one of the diseases related to tick bites: Lyme disease or Rocky Mountain spotted fever. You may see a slightly raised red spot at the point where you were bitten by the tick, with a clear area in the center—what's known as a "bull's eye" rash. If any of these symptoms develop, see a medical professional—and tell your doctor that you were bitten by a tick. Early symptoms of these diseases can mimic the flu, masking the more serious illness.

Toothache

Sometimes a piece of food becomes lodged between two teeth, sometimes a tooth is cracked or fissured, and sometimes a tooth is abscessed; all can cause toothache. Even a gum infection can lead to toothache as inflammation spreads throughout the mouth. If you have a toothache that gets worse or fails to improve with treatment, be sure to see your dentist, particularly if the pain is accompanied by an earache or a fever. A tooth infection can lead to serious complications, including an infected jawbone.

RINSE WITH HYDROGEN PEROXIDE

Rinsing your mouth with hydrogen peroxide can stop a toothache quickly and kill bacteria that could be contributing to the problem. Rinse with a tablespoon of hydrogen peroxide for at least thirty seconds, don't swallow, and then rinse your mouth again with lukewarm water.

SEA SALT SOLUTION

As with painful gums, sea salt can be a helpful solution for a toothache. Sea salt not only reduces the swelling in your gums but it also has the ability to draw bacteria and infection out of any abscesses. A sea salt solution can help relieve the worst of the pain until you can get in to see your dentist. Dissolve a teaspoon of sea salt in a cup of warm water, and swish it in your mouth for thirty seconds. Spit it out and do it again three or four times. Once you've alleviated the initial pain, continue to use this mouth rinse twice a day after you brush your teeth, to help you avoid any recurrence.

APPLY AN ASPIRIN PASTE

The salicylic acid in aspirin can help stop pain fast. Pulverize an adult aspirin and add a few drops of water to form a paste. Rub the paste onto the affected tooth, breathing through your mouth for a few minutes to give the aspirin time to work before it begins to dissolve. Try not to eat or drink anything for at least half an hour.

Urinary Tract Infection

Urinary tract infections are usually caused by bacteria that enter the urinary tract via the urethra. A painful, burning sensation upon urination, the urge to urinate even though you've just gone, and severe discomfort are the most common symptoms. If your urinary tract infection (UTI) lasts longer than two days or worsens even after using home remedies, see your doctor right away.

DRINK PURE CRANBERRY JUICE

Pure, unsweetened cranberry juice is an excellent remedy for treating urinary tract infections as soon as you notice minor discomfort. Buy at least a gallon of pure cranberry juice and start drinking about eight ounces hourly. Keep on drinking it for a few hours after the discomfort disappears to eliminate any remaining bacteria.

Why It Works Antioxidants in cranberries change the bacteria that try to cling to the walls of the urinary tract, making it difficult or impossible for them to stick. Some studies have shown that cranberries make the urinary tract walls slippery, creating a surface inhospitable to bacteria.

EAT BLUEBERRIES

While a handful of blueberries won't stave off a UTI in progress, they will help prevent the next one. Sprinkle a generous handful over your morning cereal, or add them to yogurt or ice cream. Blueberries have the same bacteria-killing properties as cranberries. Although cranberry juice might be easier to procure than blueberry juice, a refreshing smoothie made with blueberries may be just the thing to ease the discomfort of a UTI.

BEAT BACTERIA WITH BAKING SODA

To help prevent a urinary tract infection from worsening, blend one teaspoon of baking soda with eight ounces of water and drink it quickly. The baking soda alkalizes your urine, helping to prevent bacteria from multiplying. Repeat this hourly for up to four hours.

Vaginal Dryness

If you've been through menopause and you have sexual relations, you may find that the changes in your body include vaginal dryness. This is a normal condition in women over fifty-five, but it can make sex painful—or at least uncomfortable—and can limit your potential for sexual satisfaction. The lubricants you buy over the counter may not correct the problem well enough or long enough for your situation.

COCONUT OIL

This easy-to-use remedy, applied to the woman's genital area just before sex, can restore lubrication temporarily and ease the process of intercourse. While it appears solid in the jar, coconut oil turns to a liquid as it warms up, and it's harmless to vaginal tissue. It also has the added bonus of antibacterial qualities—and it's edible.

OLIVE OIL

Equally effective and a healthy alternative to petroleum-based or estrogen-based lubricants, olive oil applied directly to the vaginal area will provide the necessary lubrication for intercourse. It lasts longer than some over-the-counter lubricants because it's not water soluble. That being said, you may want to place a towel under you during sex, as olive oil can stain your sheets permanently.

ALOE

You will find personal lubricants available commercially that are made with aloe, the natural product of the aloe vera plant. Look for products that have at least 90 percent organic aloe. These clean up easily after sex, and they stay slippery during intercourse so that you can enjoy the entire experience.

Varicose Veins

Varicose veins are enlarged veins that can be seen bulging through the skin's surface, typically in the lower legs and feet.

ELEVATE YOUR LEGS

Because varicose veins are often damaged, they can throb uncomfortably. Elevate your legs while sitting to ease the discomfort. Wearing support hose can help prevent throbbing and ease swelling.

APPLY WITCH HAZEL

Witch hazel's anti-inflammatory properties can help ease the discomfort of varicose veins. Use undiluted witch hazel, which is a stronger concentration than what you typically find in the plastic bottle in the drugstore. Simply cleanse the affected area with soap and water before applying the witch hazel with a cotton pad. There is no need to rinse afterward.

FLEX YOUR FEET

When seated for long periods of time, improve circulation and prevent discomfort by flexing your feet up and down as if you are pressing and releasing your car's brakes. You can also rotate your feet and swing them back and forth to encourage blood to keep moving through your legs. Be sure to get up and walk for at least five minutes each hour. This will help keep blood from pooling and prevent varicose veins from worsening.

Warts

Warts are small, lumpy growths that are caused by the human papilloma virus (HPV). When you get a wart on your finger, it's called a "common" wart, while a wart on the bottom of your foot is a "plantar" wart. Basically, these two kinds of warts are the same thing. Although they often fall off on their own eventually, they are unsightly and can be itchy. A dermatologist can remove a wart in a minute or two, but the process may be costly and often is not covered by health insurance.

DISSOLVE IT WITH WHITE VINEGAR

The acid in white vinegar can dissolve a wart in as little as two weeks. Simply soak a cotton ball with white vinegar and attach it to your wart with tape or a bandage. Repeat daily until the wart disappears.

ERASE IT WITH ALOE VERA GEL

Aloe vera gel contains malic acid, which is capable of dissolving a wart. Dip a cotton ball in aloe gel and attach it to your wart with tape or a bandage. Repeat daily until the wart disappears.

CRUSH IT WITH GARLIC

A study published in the *International Journal of Dermatology* confirmed what old wives have known for centuries: Garlic applied directly to a wart will kill and remove the wart within two weeks. Garlic contains natural antifungal and antibacterial agents that can relieve many kinds of illnesses.

1. Wash your hands thoroughly with soap and water.
2. Peel a clove of garlic, and cut it in half.
3. Gently rub the wart with the cut side of the garlic to coat it with natural garlic juices. Continue to rub it with garlic for up to two minutes.

4. Using athletic tape, adhere the other half of the garlic clove to your wart, with the cut side against the wart. The piece of garlic should be a little larger than the wart itself.
5. Leave the garlic in place overnight. You can remove it in the morning and expose the wart to the air, but repeat the process at night.
6. Continue to do this until the wart is gone. You may see the wart become discolored as the process continues; this is an indication that it's dying. The whole process may take up to two weeks.

Water Retention

Water retention is an abnormal accumulation of liquid in the body, including the circulatory system, organs, and other tissues. Symptoms include swollen feet and legs, swollen arms and hands, and in some cases, swelling in other parts of the body.

REDUCE YOUR SALT INTAKE

Give up the salty snacks, salted nuts, fast food, soda pop, and other foods and drinks that add large amounts of sodium to your body. Salt's role in your body chemistry is to retain fluid, so if there's a lot of salt in your diet and you feel blown up like a beach ball, it's doing its job. Reducing the junk food and sodium-rich drinks in your diet will help all that extra water find its way out.

BANISH BLOATING WITH BANANAS

Bananas are high in potassium, which is essential in battling water retention. Eat them plain, slice them onto your cereal, or make a smoothie. Have at least three bananas in three hours to quickly elevate your potassium level.

DRINK CRANBERRY JUICE

Cranberries contain natural diuretic compounds. Drink pure cranberry juice regularly to help flush your system and eliminate water retention. Be sure to drink plenty of water, too; staying hydrated is one of the best ways to keep your system balanced and functioning properly.

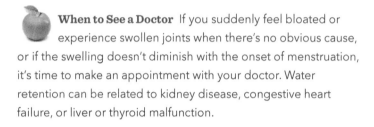 **When to See a Doctor** If you suddenly feel bloated or experience swollen joints when there's no obvious cause, or if the swelling doesn't diminish with the onset of menstruation, it's time to make an appointment with your doctor. Water retention can be related to kidney disease, congestive heart failure, or liver or thyroid malfunction.

Yeast Infection

Yeast infections occur when benign yeast called *Candida albicans* multiply, causing itching and redness. In many cases, white discharge and a foul odor accompany other symptoms. If a yeast infection persists for more than three days or becomes worse at any point, consult your doctor immediately to rule out a more serious problem.

STAY DRY AND BREATHABLE

Give up your sexy nylon or spandex underwear and replace them with white cotton—or at least with panties that have a white cotton liner. Panty hose and tights can exacerbate an existing yeast infection and create an environment for your next one, so choose hose and tights with a cotton-lined panty. After you shower, dry your vulva with a blow dryer set on low to keep new yeast from finding the warm, moist area they crave.

APPLY YOGURT

Buy a cup of plain nonfat yogurt with live, active cultures. Dip a tampon in the yogurt and insert it into the vagina. Leave it in place for thirty minutes; then remove it and discard it. Repeat this treatment four times each day for up to three days.

DOUCHE WITH WHITE VINEGAR

Combine two tablespoons of white vinegar with one quart of distilled water. Douche with the entire recipe. Repeat this treatment twice daily for two days.

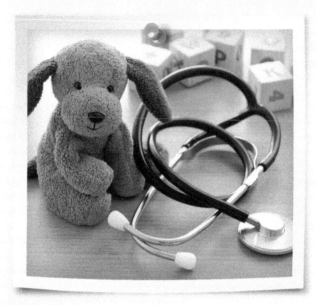

PRENATAL, BABY, AND CHILD-AGE AILMENTS

Prenatal Ailments
- Backache
- Constipation
- Fainting/ Dizziness
- Heartburn
- Hemorrhoids
- Insomnia
- Leg Cramps
- Mood Swings
- Morning Sickness/Nausea
- Oral Health

Baby Ailments
- Colds
- Colic
- Constipation
- Cradle Cap
- Diaper Rash
- Diarrhea
- Eczema
- Fever
- Teething

Child Ailments
- Asthma
- Chicken Pox
- Colds
- Constipation
- Croup

- Diarrhea
- Ear Infection
- Fever
- Flu
- Hand, Foot, and Mouth Disease (Coxsackie Virus)
- Headache
- Head Lice
- Pinkeye (Conjunctivitis)
- Sore Throat
- Stomachache

CHAPTER 7

Prenatal, Baby, and Child-Age Ailments

At no time in your life is what you do for your health more important than during a pregnancy. Every substance, chemical, and nutrient you take in will have an effect on your growing baby. You need to take more care than ever before to maintain the safest and purest standards you possibly can as your body assembles a new central nervous system for your unborn child. This usually means that over-the-counter and prescription medications are not available to you—so home remedies become a useful and effective part of your health care. Because essential oils can have powerful effects, especially when used undiluted or directly on the skin, they are not included in the remedies in this section, as they should not be used on babies, children, or by women who are pregnant or breastfeeding.

Once your baby arrives, you still have the option of choosing natural health-care methods over pharmaceuticals—and many of these methods are recommended by doctors. Some illnesses do require antibiotics or specialized medications to return your baby to good health, but in many cases, the common ailments that trouble babies can be treated with the same remedies our grandmothers and great-grandmothers may have used to soothe their children when they were small.

As your baby becomes a toddler, a number of common issues can be solved using natural means and simple solutions. Remember that high fevers, significant problems with breathing, sports injuries, and other serious conditions still require a doctor's intervention, but a tummy ache or sore throat may be treated just as well with an herbal or natural remedy as by a prescription. You may be able to bring your child relief much faster than waiting for a doctor's schedule to open up, and you can avoid unpleasant side effects that sometimes accompany prescription drugs.

Prenatal Ailments

Backache

As your baby grows, your center of gravity shifts and your weight increases, two factors that cause backache in most pregnant women. In addition, your body produces a hormone called relaxin, which allows the ligaments in your pelvic region to relax as the time for childbirth approaches. Two sheets of muscles in your back separate as your uterus expands, making lower back pain your constant companion.

EXERCISE TO STRENGTHEN MUSCLES

While you may feel like you can't move, movement is the best thing for your back pain. Take a walk every day, or try swimming, an exercise that relieves the pain of carrying so much extra weight by making that weight buoyant. The more you can stretch the muscles that hurt, the more flexibility you will have. This eases the pain.

ICE AND FIRE

Try putting an ice pack (or a bag of frozen vegetables) wrapped in a towel on the area in pain, for an interval of twenty minutes, three or four times a day. After several days of this treatment, switch to a heating pad on the area where the pain is centered. Keep the heat on your back, not your abdomen—you don't want to heat the baby's area.

YOGA FOR FLEXIBILITY

Stretching in slow, gentle ways can do wonders for back pain, and it can soothe other aching muscles and help you keep your balance. Take a prenatal yoga class or perform the poses using a video or other visual aid. Yoga needs to be done correctly to get the maximum benefit, so get the guidance you need to get started.

Constipation

Half of all pregnant women experience some difficulty with constipation. Your body produces more progesterone, a hormone that relaxes muscles—and some of those muscles are in your intestines, so they process food more slowly than normal. If you're taking an iron supplement, it could be making your constipation worse, as well.

HIGH FIBER FOR SMOOTHER MOVEMENT

Fruits, vegetables, and whole grains—all things you should be eating anyway—can help your digestive system stay on track by providing the fiber your body needs. If you are already eating these foods and you're still struggling, add a tablespoon or two of wheat bran to your morning cereal.

WATER, WATER EVERYWHERE

Drink lots of water to give your intestines the lubrication they need to function more easily. Carry a water bottle with you wherever you go, and strive for sixty-four to forty-eight ounces a day.

KEEP MOVING

Exercise can make a big difference in the way your body handles all kinds of issues—pain, stress, constipation, digestion, and many others. In this case, more movement keeps your intestines functioning properly, while spending most of your time sitting can aggravate your constipation. Walking, swimming, and yoga are all excellent choices during a pregnancy.

Fainting/Dizziness

If the room fades away for a few seconds when you stand up quickly, or if you start to feel lightheaded while you've been on your feet for a while, you are experiencing a normal, if disquieting, symptom of pregnancy. Blood struggles to get all the way to your brain when you're pregnant, especially if you've been standing up for a long time. Your uterus also demands a great deal of blood to protect and nourish your growing infant.

SIT DOWN

It may seem like an obvious point, but it's worth saying: Do your best to avoid standing up for long periods. If you're out shopping, take breaks by stopping in a coffee shop and having a cup of tea, or sit down on a bench and enjoy some people watching.

SHIFT YOUR WEIGHT

Keep your blood circulating by shifting your weight from one leg to the other so it won't pool in your legs and feet. When you're standing, try not to lock your knees, as this also reduces blood flow.

KEEP DRINKING

Letting yourself become dehydrated can bring on dizziness and even fainting. Drink plenty of fluids, even though this will mean that you'll be looking for the bathroom more often. Your blood moves through your body more easily when you have plenty of water in your system.

Heartburn

When you're pregnant, your body produces more hormones, with progesterone leading the pack. Progesterone relaxes muscles throughout your body in preparation for childbirth, even the ones that are not directly involved in the birthing process. One of these is the valve at the entrance to the stomach. This valve normally keeps stomach acid out of the esophagus. Add the pressure of your baby pushing on your stomach, and you've got painful heartburn.

EAT SMALL MEALS

You have to eat for nutrition for you and your baby, and chances are you're hungry all the time. Try eating smaller meals more frequently to give you body less to digest at one time.

A GLASS OF MILK BEFORE BED

It's the most basic of heartburn remedies, but a glass of milk before you lie down for the night can help neutralize stomach acid.

EASY ON THE FAT

Fatty foods—like French fries, cheeseburgers, or deep-fried anything— are hard to digest, and they can cause heartburn even when you're not pregnant. Stick to whole grains, lean meats, and fruits and vegetables.

Hemorrhoids

Progesterone, the hormone that relaxes muscles in advance of childbirth, is at work in your anus as well as in your reproductive system. When your muscles relax, the varicose veins in your rectal region swell and become uncomfortable. Bearing down to pass bowel movements can make this condition worse.

TRY TISSUE SALTS

Tissue salts, the twelve minerals found in the human body, were discovered in the nineteenth century by a German doctor who analyzed the cremated remains of hundreds of patients. Homeopaths believe that replacing these minerals in the body can help regulate processes that have gone awry; some say that hemorrhoids will be reduced in as little as a day or two. At worst, nothing will happen—these naturally occurring substances are harmless. They come in pill or tablet form.

A DAB OF WITCH HAZEL

Witch hazel is a natural anti-inflammatory that is used in many ointments and astringent products. Saturate a cotton ball with witch hazel tincture, and place it on the affected area. Keep it there overnight, and repeat this for another night or two. (You can also buy medicated wipes that contain witch hazel.) In most cases, the swelling and pain will disappear in two to three days.

Why It Works Witch hazel contains tannins, molecules that encourage the proteins in your skin to bond with one another. This process reduces inflammation and promotes healing, making witch hazel a good option for treating bug bites, eczema, and other skin conditions as well as hemorrhoids.

NATURAL IRON TONIC

A number of iron supplements cause constipation, which in turn causes hemorrhoids to flare up and become painful. Instead of using iron supplements in pill form, look for the liquid option, also known as Floradix. This plant-based tonic is absorbed into the body more easily than synthetic pills, and it does not cause constipation. A number of manufacturers make a liquid iron supplement and combine it with other minerals and herbs, so check the labels to see what may be included in the one you choose.

Insomnia

BabyCenter notes that eight out of every ten pregnant women have trouble sleeping. So many factors work against your sleep: the discomfort of changes in your body's shape, the need to urinate several times during the night, leg cramps, and feelings of anxiety about your baby's safe and healthy gestation.

DON'T WATCH THE CLOCK

If you aren't asleep in twenty to thirty minutes after getting into bed, get up again. Go into a different room and read, watch TV, listen to music, and get your mind off whatever's keeping you awake. When you feel drowsy again, go back to bed. Staying in bed and watching the minutes tick away only increases anxiety and discomfort.

TRY RELAXATION TECHNIQUES

Deep breathing, progressive muscle relaxation, and guided imagery are all excellent techniques for calming your body and mind at bedtime (and any time). Your midwife or obstetrician may be able to help you learn these, or you may find a health club or YMCA in your area that has classes in these techniques for pregnant women.

CUT THE CAFFEINE

If you haven't given up caffeine during your pregnancy, limit your use of it to the morning. Afternoon and evening caffeine will keep anyone awake at night, whether or not they're pregnant.

WATCH OUT FOR SPICES

Heavy, spicy food for dinner can cause indigestion later, and heartburn when you're lying down and trying to digest at night. Either of these will keep you awake.

REDUCE FLUIDS AT NIGHT

You need to take in fluids throughout the day, but if frequent bathroom trips are keeping you up at night, it may be advisable to cut down on fluids toward the day's end.

Leg Cramps

That sharp pain that wakes you in the middle of the night usually happens in your feet, calves, or thighs, and it's enough to have you out of bed and on your feet in seconds. While findings are inconclusive, doctors believe that cramps come from reduced levels of calcium and magnesium in your body during pregnancy, because your baby is using these nutrients.

FLEX YOUR FEET

Flexing and pointing your feet can release a cramp fairly quickly, and walking can help, as well. When you flex your foot, you straighten and stretch the muscles in your calves and the backs of your thighs (hamstrings). Pointing your toes stretches muscles in your shins and your quadriceps in your upper legs.

MASSAGE AND EXERCISE WORK

Have your partner massage your feet, calves, or thighs to release the muscles. During the day, get a good walk in to keep these muscles flexible, wearing sneakers or other low-heeled shoes.

TALK TO YOUR DOCTOR ABOUT SUPPLEMENTS

If your cramps happen frequently and they're keeping you up at night, your doctor can recommend a calcium and magnesium supplement to increase these nutrients in your body, so you'll have enough for your baby and for you.

Mood Swings

You've always been a stable, calm, even-tempered person, but now that you're in your first or third trimester of pregnancy, you suddenly catch yourself crying at fast-food commercials and going into a panic attack at the mall. It may not feel normal, but it's actually very common during pregnancy, especially toward the end when hormonal changes are at their peak.

GO WITH THE FLOW

Your changes in mood and temperament are beyond your control, but you can take control by recognizing these sudden swings for what they are. Do your best to remain nonjudgmental about yourself. Your feelings are real, and they are part of this experience of creating a new life. Face these changes and practice relaxation techniques to get past the worst of them.

BUILD UP YOUR OMEGA-3S

Your baby needs omega-3 fatty acids to build a new brain, so all of these important nutrients in your body are called on to complete the task. This can leave you feeling moody and depressed—and the sleeplessness, back pain, and other symptoms you feel all pile onto your sense of well-being. Taking an omega-3 supplement (with your doctor's guidance) can help. If you don't want to swallow a pill, increase the fish in your diet—especially salmon and halibut.

TAKE A WALK

You'll hear this over and over throughout your pregnancy: Exercise can be a remedy for a wide range of uncomfortable symptoms. Taking a brisk walk can raise your endorphin levels, which automatically elevates your mood. If you can't get out to walk, keep a yoga video handy for your next break.

Morning Sickness/Nausea

As many as 90 percent of pregnant women experience morning sickness, but knowing this fact doesn't make your experience any less miserable. The symptoms usually disappear by the second trimester, through not for everyone—and maintaining proper nutritional levels can be difficult when you're constantly nauseated and/or vomiting.

SNACK AT NIGHT

Keep healthy munchies by your bed—such as trail mix and granola— and have a snack before you go to sleep. This will keep you from waking up on a completely empty stomach, one of the conditions that leads to morning sickness.

GET SOME GINGER

Scientific studies have shown that ginger has a remarkable ability to settle the stomach and quell nausea. Drink real ginger ale or ginger tea, eat ginger snaps, or try candied ginger. Make sure that the ginger in whatever you eat is real, not an artificial flavoring.

Why It Works *Obstetric and Gynecology International* reported in 2013 that ginger was more effective than a placebo in relieving nausea during pregnancy. While studies show ginger's effectiveness, scientists are uncertain of the reason behind it—though it may be connected with the gingerols and shogaols that give ginger its pungent taste.

CHOOSE APPEALING FOODS

So you'd like to get plenty of iron and vitamin A, but right now spinach turns your stomach. Choose other foods that appeal to you, and keep striving to take in the nutrients you need—but on your terms. Avoid spicy or fatty foods, both of which can increase your digestive discomfort, and stick to fruits, vegetables, and whole grains that don't turn your stomach when you look at them.

Oral Health

The hormones that cause all the other changes described in this chapter also affect your teeth and gums—specifically, the way your gums react to plaque. You may experience a condition that dentists call "pregnancy gingivitis," causing swollen, tender, reddened gums. You may think that you can just tough this out until your baby is born, but research shows that this gingivitis is linked to preterm, low-birth-weight babies.

INCREASE VITAMINS C

Research shows that vitamin C improved gums' natural defense mechanisms against plaque buildup. Too little vitamin C can lead to loose teeth and bleeding gums. If you need to increase your intake of vitamin C beyond the prenatal vitamins you may be taking, try sweet potatoes, citrus fruits, and red peppers.

IF YOU CAN'T BRUSH

If the thought of putting a toothbrush in your mouth makes you nauseated, use an antiplaque or fluoride mouthwash, and rinse your mouth at least twice a day. This will loosen the plaque and help you keep your gums clear. A baking soda solution of one teaspoon of baking soda in one cup of water can serve as an acid-neutralizing mouthwash, especially if you are vomiting regularly.

SEE YOUR DENTIST

Once you can handle having your dental hygienist's hands in your mouth, see your dentist regularly for cleanings. Basic hygiene visits can keep the plaque buildup under control.

When to See a Doctor Some pregnant women develop tumors in their mouths—noncancerous inflammations that appear when gums are irritated and swollen. These will shrink and disappear after your baby is born, but if the tumors are interfering with your ability to chew or swallow, you may need to have them removed. Talk to your dentist about any issues you have with painful gums or tumors.

Baby Ailments

Colds

The American Academy of Pediatrics warns that over-the-counter medications aren't safe for children under two years old, and they may be harmful or even ineffective for children under six. With this in mind, many parents now look to natural remedies and simple solutions to ease a baby's discomfort during a cold.

THE WONDERS OF STEAM

Moist air helps loosen your baby's congestion and makes it easier for your little one to breathe. A cool-mist vaporizer or humidifier will do the trick, but in a pinch, try steaming up your bathroom by turning on the shower and running hot water.

SALINE DROPS

You can make your own saline drops at home, our buy an over-the-counter preparation that's safe for babies. If you prefer to make your own, here's how to do it:

1. Dissolve ½ teaspoon of salt in 8 ounces of warm water. You can store this in a glass jar for about 24 hours, but it will start to grow bacteria after that.
2. Lay your baby on his back with a folded or rolled towel behind his neck so that his head is angled slightly back and his nostrils are pointing up. Using a bulb syringe, squeeze 2 or 3 drops of saline solution into each nostril. This will loosen the congestion. Wait 20 to 30 seconds, and try to keep your baby's head still during that time.
3. Squeeze any remaining solution out of the bulb syringe, and then insert the tip into the baby's nostril. Release the bulb slowly to suck out the saline solution and mucus. Remove the syringe and squeeze its contents into a tissue. Discard the tissue.
4. Repeat this with the other nostril. When you are finished, wash the syringe in mild soap and water.
5. Repeat these steps several times throughout the day, but not any more frequently than that. Saline solution will dry out a baby's nose after a few days of use.

CHICKEN SOUP

If your baby is older than six months, warm chicken broth is remarkably effective in helping to relieve congestion and speed a cold's resolution. After all the hype from generations of mothers, scientists have studied the healing power of chicken soup and have found it to be very real. If your baby isn't ready for soup, warmed apple juice or even warm water can help.

Colic

Here's the definition of colic: Uncontrollable crying in an otherwise healthy baby younger than five months, with crying for more than three hours in a row on three or more days in a week, for three weeks. It's not an illness, and it won't cause any long-term harm, but it can be maddening for you and certainly uncomfortable for your baby.

IT'S THE MOTION

A rocking chair or a baby swing can help soothe a crying baby. If your baby doesn't respond to these, try carrying your baby in a front pack or a sling, so she can hear your heart beating and your voice close by. Some babies quiet down when they ride in the car, so try taking a drive with your baby secured in her carrier in the backseat.

WARM WATER

Warm (not hot) water in a water bottle can help calm a baby. Use a hot water bottle and fill it with warm water, but not so warm that it feels hot to your touch. Babies have new skin with a low tolerance for heat and cold. Wrap the bottle in a towel and put it on your stomach, and hold your baby on top of it. If this doesn't work, a warm bath can help relax and calm a colicky baby.

SWADDLING IS SOOTHING

Your baby recently emerged from a very cozy place inside you, and now the world is large, bright, drafty, and potentially scary. Swaddling—wrapping the baby in a manner that feels snug and safe—can restore your baby's sense of security, which may quiet her cries.

WHITE NOISE SOUNDS LIKE MOMMY

While she was in the womb, your baby heard your heartbeat and other pleasant, whooshing or gurgling noises. Now the world is full of sudden noises, unfamiliar voices, and unnatural sounds. Your house is full of white noisemakers, however—the washer and dryer, the dishwasher, the exhaust fan in the kitchen, the vacuum cleaner, or even a recording of waves or wind sounds. Any of these may remind your baby of those sounds she heard before the world became so huge and noisy.

Constipation

It's hard to tell if your baby is actually constipated, or if he has not yet established a natural rhythm and pattern for his bowel movements. If your baby passes hard, dry stools or does not have a bowel movement for three days or more, he may be struggling with constipation.

SWITCH FORMULA BRANDS

If you're feeding your baby with formula, there may be something in the formula that's causing constipation. Talk with your pediatrician about choosing a different brand. (Sometimes adding a teaspoon of corn syrup to the formula can offer the needed boost.) Research shows that breast-fed babies are rarely constipated because breast milk contains exactly the right balance of fat and nutrients. If breastfeeding is an option for you, you may want to try it.

SWITCH SOLID FOODS

Many babies become constipated when they begin eating solid food, because the initial foods babies eat can be shy on fiber (rice cereal, for example, has almost no fiber). Try adding pureed prunes, pears, or apricots to your baby's diet.

EXERCISE CAN HELP

If your baby is too young to crawl, try making bicycle motions with her legs while she's lying on her back. This can be all the additional movement she needs to get her intestines in gear. If she can crawl, try encouraging her to crawl for longer distances.

When to See a Doctor If your baby's anus bleeds after a bowel movement, talk with your doctor about changing her diet. Bleeding is likely a sign of an anal fissure, a tear around the anal opening. While it's easily treated with a dab of lotion or aloe vera, also consult your doctor.

Cradle Cap

Does your baby have dandruff? That flaky, dry skin on top of his head may look like dandruff, but it's actually a condition called seborrheic dermatitis, and it's more unsightly than it is dangerous. The flaky skin may be accompanied by oily patches, yellow or brown scaling, or crusty areas. Symptoms may appear on eyebrows, eyelids, or as far down as in the armpits. Doctors don't know what causes cradle cap, but it is not a sign of bad hygiene.

TRY A NATURAL OIL

You don't actually need to do anything at all about cradle cap—it will clear up on its own in a few months—but if you just can't stand to look at it, try rubbing a little natural oil into your baby's scalp. Almond or olive oil is good for this. Leave the oil on for about fifteen minutes, and then use a baby comb or brush to (very gently) remove the flakes that have been loosened. Wash out the oil with a baby shampoo.

BABY SHAMPOO MAY DO IT

Many sources say that daily shampooing with a soap formulated for babies' heads is the best way to reduce cradle cap.

COCONUT OIL WORKS

Put a little bit of coconut oil on the affected areas at night before bed, and brush or wash it out in the morning. Not only does it smell good but also moisturizes nicely.

Diaper Rash

Diaper rash is caused by excess moisture, and complications can occur when a baby's diaper is allowed to remain in place after he or she has soiled it. Despite your most diligent efforts, your baby may still get diaper rash, which is red, itchy, and often quite painful.

BATHE IN BAKING SODA AND OATMEAL

The soothing properties of baking soda and oatmeal can relieve your baby's discomfort.

1. At the first sign of a rash, give your baby a bath in a basin that contains 2 gallons of warm water and 1 heaping tablespoon of baking soda.
2. Be sure the affected area is covered by the water, and try to keep him or her occupied for 10 minutes so the baking soda has time to work.
3. Remove your baby from the bath, empty the water, and replace it with another 2 gallons of warm water that has ½ cup of plain, unflavored oatmeal in it.
4. Keep your baby in this bath for another 10 minutes; then rinse baby's body and make sure no bits of oatmeal remain.
5. Dry your baby, apply a thick layer of diaper rash ointment, and put on a clean diaper.

Why It Works Oatmeal contains polysaccharides, a complex carbohydrate that forms a gel when mixed with water. This soothing gel protects the skin from outside elements, softening dry skin and taking the itch out of chicken pox and rashes.

SOOTHE WITH COCONUT OIL

If you're all out of diaper rash ointment and need a barrier cream to keep wetness away from baby's tender skin, coconut oil will do the trick. Wash and dry your baby and apply a thick layer of coconut oil before diapering. Reapply as needed, even after the diaper rash disappears.

DUST WITH CORNSTARCH

You can treat a baby's diaper rash with cornstarch by simply dusting the affected area with cornstarch after cleansing it thoroughly. Change the baby's diaper as soon as it is soiled. Repeat the process to keep moisture away from the skin and promote healing.

Diarrhea

Just as it's hard to tell if your baby is constipated, diarrhea may also be a mystery. Babies have loose stools as a matter of course, but if you see a major change—more watery stools or a change in volume, for example—there may be something out of the ordinary going on: a viral or bacterial infection, a food allergy, or just something that didn't agree with his tummy.

GIVE SOLID FOOD

If your baby is eating solid food already, go ahead and feed him his usual diet of whole grains, meats, yogurt, fruit, and vegetables. These will help restore normalcy in his digestive system.

GIVE PLENTY OF LIQUIDS

The biggest hazard to babies with diarrhea is dehydration, which can lead to more serious health issues. A pediatric electrolyte solution may be the best choice, as the sugary juices and soft drinks you *might* think are easier on the stomach can actually make diarrhea worse. Sugar draws water into the intestines, increasing stool softness.

USE THE BRAT DIET

Bananas, rice, applesauce, and toast are the magic combination for slowing down diarrhea in people of any age.

Why It Works The BRAT diet is four bland foods without much fat, protein, or fiber—the hard-to-digest materials your child's body wants to expel through diarrhea. This is not a nutritionally sound diet, so you'll want to move your child back to normal foods as soon as possible.

When to See a Doctor If your baby vomits more than once, has bloody or black stool, or has a fever above 101 degrees, call your pediatrician. Call the doctor if you see signs of dehydration: a dry mouth, no urination for six hours, or crying without tears.

Eczema

If your child is going to have the skin rash known as eczema, it will appear before the age of five, most likely on your baby's scalp or cheeks. Once it appears, it may spread to the arms, chest, or other parts of the body. The tendency toward eczema is inherited, so if you had it as a child, it's likely your child will have it, as well. This itchy skin condition can be very uncomfortable for babies, especially because scratching can cause scarring or infection.

BATHE AND MOISTURIZE

While the common wisdom is that it's not good to bathe a baby every day, a daily bath may actually be better for a baby with eczema. Use water that's not too warm, and don't allow your baby to sit in a pool of soapy water. Use a hypoallergenic soap or a baby cleanser that isn't soap, and dry the baby by patting him with a towel as soon as you're through with the bath. While the baby's skin is still damp, apply a moisturizer—an ointment will seal in more moisture than a lotion can.

TREAT THE ITCH

The best way to keep your baby from scratching an itch is to make that itch go away. Use cool compresses several times a day, pressed gently on the affected area. Choose clothing made with natural fabrics (cotton), and avoid any garments that are scratchy or irritating.

THE WONDERS OF BLEACH

Add two teaspoons of household bleach to one gallon of your baby's bath water and swirl it in before you place your baby in the tub. Make sure he doesn't drink the water! A quick rinse in plain water after the bath will take care of the chlorine smell. Pediatricians don't recommend using bleach water on the face; instead, apply petroleum jelly to affected areas on the cheeks and scalp.

Why It Works In 2009, a study published in the journal *Pediatrics* tested a number of treatments for children with eczema, and discovered that two teaspoons of bleach per gallon of bath water was five times more effective in treating eczema than plain water.

Fever

Everyone's temperature rises toward the end of the day and drops again overnight, so a warm forehead in the evening does not necessarily mean that your baby is running a fever. When your baby seems listless, doesn't want to play, and doesn't eat, however, she may be fighting off an infection that spikes her temperature well above normal. The general agreement among pediatricians is that normal temperature for a baby ranges from 97 degrees to 100.3 degrees Fahrenheit.

WATCH FOR BEHAVIORAL CHANGES

If your baby is behaving perfectly normally despite her elevated temperature, your best course of action may be no action at all. As long as your baby is eating, drinking, and playing the way she always does, the fever is not making her uncomfortable enough to change what she's doing. She may fight off whatever low-grade infection she has without assistance.

SPONGE BATH

Giving your baby a sponge bath with lukewarm (not hot or cold) water can help cool down a fever. Never give your baby a bath using rubbing alcohol—this can be absorbed through the skin and be harmful to her.

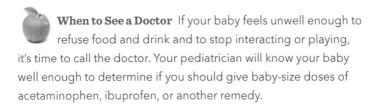 **When to See a Doctor** If your baby feels unwell enough to refuse food and drink and to stop interacting or playing, it's time to call the doctor. Your pediatrician will know your baby well enough to determine if you should give baby-size doses of acetaminophen, ibuprofen, or another remedy.

Teething

Every baby grows teeth, and the process of bringing those first teeth out in the open can be painful and uncomfortable for your baby. Luckily, there is a wide range of solutions that can help you make the transition easier. Baby ibuprofen or acetaminophen will help, but many parents would prefer a non-medicinal approach.

COLD FOODS HELP

Give your baby chilled foods like applesauce, yogurt, or pudding to help with the discomfort of teething. Frozen fruit can be a good choice—let your baby suck or gnaw on a piece of fruit, but makes sure to put the fruit in a mesh bag to keep it from becoming a choking hazard.

CHILL A TEETHING RING

You can find a teething ring with fluid in it in your favorite baby-items retailer. These magical rings go into the refrigerator for an hour and come out ready for your baby to chew to his heart's content. The ring is large enough that you can hold onto it if your baby cannot.

RUB THE GUMS

Use your finger to rub your baby's gums firmly enough to trick his brain into forgetting about the pain. When you rub for a moment or two, your finger will squeak against the gum, a sensation and sound your baby is likely to love.

Child Ailments

Asthma

If your child coughs persistently at night, has difficulty breathing, or if you can hear wheezing when he breathes, he has the symptoms of childhood asthma. Some children do not have these symptoms on a daily basis, but they have severe attacks of asthma when they are around triggers: seasonal pollen, cigarette smoke, campfire smoke, perfumes, pet dander, or large quantities of dust. There is no cure for this condition, but it can be controlled with the use of medical intervention. Home remedies should be used in conjunction with medical solutions such as inhaled medications.

ELIMINATE FUR AND FEATHERS

One of the best things you can do for your asthmatic child is to remove any pets that have fur or feathers, especially dogs, cats, or birds. This may be difficult for your child and you, but pet dander (the dry skin that flakes off pets) is one of the top asthma triggers. Once your pet has found a new home, dust and vacuum your home and wash any pillowcases, bedspreads, rugs, curtains, and other cloth surfaces that may have collected pet dander.

VANQUISH MOLD

Mold is sneaky; it lurks in the dark, damp places in your home like the corners of basements, the back of a cabinet in your bathroom, and in showers and bathtubs even if you clean your house thoroughly on a regular basis. The insides of air conditioners, furnaces, and heating ducts can be home to mold spores, as well. Go through your home looking for mold, and kill it wherever you find it. You may want to have this done professionally; contact your local heating, ventilation, and air-conditioning service company for information on a whole-house purge.

Why It Works Some molds produce mycotoxins, spores that are hazardous to humans. Exposure can cause a range of symptoms, from nasal congestion to wheezing and difficulty breathing. Prolonged exposure can cause brain damage. Removing these stimuli from your home can make an enormous difference in your child's health—and your own.

UN-SCENT YOUR HOME

Those air fresheners you have plugged into your electrical sockets often spew particulates that carry scent into your home—but they are some of the most insidious asthma triggers, because they encourage you to breathe them in deeply. Scented candles, perfumed air fresheners, aerosol or pump spray scents, colognes, aftershaves, and all the other scented substances in your home may aggravate your child's asthma. Learn to love your home's natural scents.

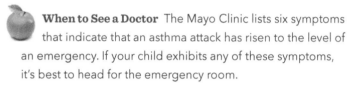

When to See a Doctor The Mayo Clinic lists six symptoms that indicate that an asthma attack has risen to the level of an emergency. If your child exhibits any of these symptoms, it's best to head for the emergency room.

1. Significant trouble breathing
2. Persistent cough or wheezing
3. No improvement even after using a rescue inhaler
4. Leaning forward in a sitting position to breathe
5. Being unable to talk without gasping
6. Peak flow meter readings in the red zone

Chicken Pox

Chicken pox is caused by a contagious virus that almost every kid gets. It starts out as a rash, after which characteristic red pockmarks develop. This disease is extremely itchy and uncomfortable, but it is important not to scratch the lesions, as this can cause the virus to spread rapidly and leave scars.

EASE WITH DIAPER RASH CREAM

Diaper rash cream contains zinc oxide, which is an astringent that helps alleviate itching and reduce swelling. Apply it liberally to the affected skin to reduce itching.

CALAMINE LOTION

Another compound that contains zinc oxide, the Calamine brand also contains phenol, which helps to cool the itchiness of chicken pox lesions. Apply it directly to each lesion with a cotton ball.

TAKE AN OATMEAL BATH

Oatmeal contains antioxidants that help to reduce inflammation and ease itching. You can buy a packaged oatmeal bath product or save money by making your own. Place one cup of uncooked oatmeal in the blender and chop the oats into a rough powder. Using a funnel, pour the oats into a dress sock or one leg of an old pair of nylons. Tie a knot in the sock or nylons just above the oats and place the sachet into a bathtub filled with very hot water. Leave it to steep for about ten minutes. Place your child into the bathtub when the temperature has cooled enough for comfort. Have the child soak in the bathtub until the water cools, and then pat dry.

Colds

Every child gets a cold now and then—in fact, the National Institutes of Health say that children get six to ten colds annually on average—but most of the remedies on the market have been found to be unsafe for very young children. The US Food and Drug Administration is still considering whether to change the guidelines on many of these over-the-counter medications for children ages two to eleven. This limits a parent's choices to home remedies, some of which can be very effective in providing temporary relief from symptoms. Whatever you use, your child will likely have the cold for seven to ten days, but you can make her feel better enough to get a good night's sleep and regain some energy.

HONEY FOR COUGHS

A teaspoon of honey for a child aged six to eleven can quiet a cough, and it can be given again if the child begins coughing again a little later. For children ages two to five, give ½ teaspoon of honey. Never give honey to a baby one year old or younger, as it can lead to infant botulism, a dangerous illness.

Why It Works A 2007 study published in *the Archives of Pediatric and Adolescent Medicine* found a small amount of honey at bedtime helped children sleep better and cough less than an over-the-counter cough suppressant. Darker honeys have more antioxidants. The viscosity of honey coats the throat and silences coughs.

SALINE FOR CONGESTION

Using a saline solution, you can relieve a child's nasal congestion. Saline is simply a cup of room-temperature water with a teaspoon of salt dissolved in it. Using a bulb syringe, place a few drops of the solution into each of your child's nostrils. Wait at least sixty seconds, and then use the bulb syringe to remove the nasal discharge. For older children, have them use the saline solution as a spray, and then blow their noses after waiting sixty seconds.

MIST FOR MOISTURE

Use a cool-mist humidifier or a vaporizer in your child's bedroom to bring more moisture into the air, making it easier to breathe by loosening congestion. When the cold has passed, be sure to clean and dry the humidifier or vaporizer and store it properly, so no moisture remains in the system and turns into mold.

Constipation

If your child is struggling to pass bowel movements, or if she hasn't gone in several days, she may be constipated. Usually, you can treat this issue at home without a doctor's intervention.

THE DRINKING CURE

Constipation can be the result of a lack of fluids in a child's system. Make sure she's drinking water, juice, or milk every day, and consider adding a glass of prune juice to the mix.

FILL UP WITH FIBER

Eating a bowl of high-fiber cereal in the morning, a sandwich on whole-grain bread for lunch, and fruits and vegetables with dinner can regulate a child's (and an adult's) digestive system and restore regularity. One cup of whole fruit and one cup of vegetables will not only ease constipation, but they also will provide your child with a nutritional boost.

TUMMY MASSAGE

Gently massage your child's belly, especially if you can feel a solid mass in her abdomen. This can help relieve stomach pain and get things moving in the right direction again.

NON-MEDICATED SUPPOSITORIES

If all else fails, you can buy glycerin suppositories over the counter at any pharmacy. These bullet-shaped capsules contain a lubricant that stimulates the rectum into working properly.

When to See a Doctor If none of these methods work for your child, it's time to seek a doctor's advice. Do not use laxatives until you have consulted with your doctor. Over-the-counter laxatives are not formulated for children; it's important to discuss all the options before employing any medication.

Croup

A common respiratory problem in young children, croup sounds much worse than it actually is. This contagious illness causes the larynx and trachea to swell and narrow, leading to an unmistakable barking cough that sounds alien enough to strike fear in a parent's heart. The child's voice gets hoarse, and he may make a crowing sound when inhaling that can make you think he cannot breathe. The symptoms usually get worse at night, when the child is lying down.

Croup will go away on its own in a few days, but your child will have significant discomfort while he has it. It's also a scary illness, so staying calm can play an important role in keeping your child from crying and increasing his difficulty breathing.

GO OUTSIDE

You may have heard stories about a panicked parent grabbing his child with croup and running outside in the middle of the night. There's a good reason to do this: The change in air temperature can relieve the airway constriction and restore your child's breathing. Some parents stumble on this solution, and then pass it on to others. It does work.

HUMID AIR WORKS, TOO

If you can't rush outside or if it's a hot night, fill your bathroom with steam and sit in there with your child for at least ten minutes. Holding your child over a humidifier and letting the moist air blow on his face can be just as effective.

FORCE FLUIDS

Keep your child hydrated with water, flavored drinks, ice pops or similar frozen treats, and slushy ice drinks. They will help to relax the airway, too.

DON'T SMOKE

No matter what respiratory issue your child has, cigarette smoke in the house will exacerbate it. Give it up, and tell any guests who smoke that this is not permitted in your house.

Diarrhea

By the time a child is out of diapers, you will have no trouble telling when a bowel movement is diarrhea. Your first line of defense against an intestinal illness is hydration, followed by foods that do not contain much fat or sugar, both because they can increase discomfort and loose stools, and because sugary foods will not replace the nutritional content your child is losing through diarrhea.

HYDRATE, HYDRATE, HYDRATE

Give your child plenty of water, or oral rehydration drinks like Pedialyte that are made to replace minerals lost during diarrhea. Sports drinks and chicken or beef bouillon are good choices, as well, because they replace the salt a child loses during an intestinal virus.

THE BRAT DIET

If your child can keep food down, you can slow loose stools by feeding her bananas, rice, applesauce, and toast. The American Academy of Pediatrics says that your children should eat a normal diet with these four foods added, as long as they can tolerate food.

THE CRAM DIET

You may have heard about another diet currently being examined by researchers. The CRAM diet replaces the bananas with cereal and the toast with milk, providing more protein and fat than the BRAT diet. Until the results of the research bear this out, you may want to add milk to your child's meals if she already drinks milk regularly.

Ear Infection

Just about every child comes down with an ear infection on occasion, most of which pass in a few days. If your child complains of ear pain or seems listless or withdrawn, there are a range of remedies to try before reaching for the phone and calling for antibiotics. If your child's ear pain is not cause by an infection—for example, if it comes from swimmer's ear or sinus pressure from allergies—try one of the remedies offered un the Earache entry in chapter 6.

HEAT IT UP

You may recall your parent using a warm water bottle, a bag of warmed salt, a warm washcloth, or even half of a warmed onion to relieve your pain when you were little. Heat is a viable and effective remedy for ear pain. Place a small bag of kosher salt or dried beans in your microwave and heat it for about twenty seconds (more or less depending on the wattage of your appliance), and then place it gently on your child's ear. Hold it there for about ten minutes. Your child may feel considerable relief in a short time.

WARM OIL

A number of oils can help to provide relief from pain. Have your child lie on her side with the affected ear up. Place two or three drops of room-temperature sesame oil, olive oil, or tea tree oil in the ear canal, and wait ten minutes. Gently place a cotton ball over (not in) the ear, and have the child sit up. The oil will drain out onto the cotton ball.

Why It Works Warm (body temperature) oil makes gentle contact with the inflamed eardrum and soothes the swollen tissue, lessening the pain and reducing the swelling. The viscosity of the oil makes it a better choice than water or another warmed liquid.

MASSAGE

You can stimulate the draining of ear fluids and release pressure by using gentle massage around the head and jaw. Pediatrician Aviva Romm recommends that you massage in a downward direction behind the ear, and "apply gentle inward pressure in front of the ear toward the cheek."

 When to See a Doctor If you child's pain is severe or if he spikes a high fever, it's time to call your pediatrician. Also watch for a yellow or white discharge from the ear, loss of appetite, or if your child cannot sleep because of pain and discomfort.

Fever

When your child has a fever and you don't have any acetaminophen or ibuprofen available, you do have other options available to you. Remember that a fever is the body's way of fighting off infection, so elevated temperature is not always a bad thing—but your child can become dehydrated while feverish.

COOL CLOTH

A cool, damp washcloth on your child's forehead can help bring temperature down, especially if your child does not feel well enough to want to move around and play. If he can stay still and keep the cloth on his head, it will help him feel better.

CHILL FROM THE INSIDE

Encourage your child to drink cool water or other fluids, and try to tempt him with ice pops, slushy drinks, and other cold favorites.

UNBUNDLE YOUR CHILD

It's a natural instinct to want to wrap your child up in extra clothing and blankets when he's sick, but you need to allow heat to escape to bring down the fever. Dress him in a layer of cotton clothing or pajamas, and keep the blankets to a minimum. If he has a chill, add a blanket until he warms up again.

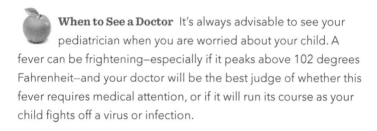 **When to See a Doctor** It's always advisable to see your pediatrician when you are worried about your child. A fever can be frightening—especially if it peaks above 102 degrees Fahrenheit—and your doctor will be the best judge of whether this fever requires medical attention, or if it will run its course as your child fights off a virus or infection.

Flu

The multiple symptoms of influenza go beyond the common cold, adding muscle aches, sore throat, and fever as well as congestion and coughing. The flu will run its course in a week or so, but in the meantime, your child can be pretty miserable—and very contagious. It's a good idea to line up your home defenses against the flu before it arrives.

DRINK PLENTY OF FLUIDS

Nothing beats congestion and mucus like fluids, so be ready with water, fruit juices, pediatric hydration drinks (like Pedialyte), and herbal teas. Caffeine isn't the best choice, because it's a natural diuretic—making your child lose as much fluid as she takes in.

FROZEN FRUIT JUICE BARS

Eating ice-pop frozen treats made with 100 percent fruit juice or pureed fruit can provide your child with nutritional value as well as hydration—and these can soothe a sore throat. Grape, strawberry, and coconut are favorites with a lot of children.

STEAM OPEN AIRWAYS

Bring a pot of water to a boil, so it produces lots of steam. Remove it from the stove and place it on a trivet or cork hot pad on your table. Have your child close his eyes and lean his face over the pot, and drape a towel gently over his head. Have him breathe deeply through his nose for up to thirty seconds. He can come out from under the tent, cool off, and repeat this treatment several times to open nasal passages. Adding a few drops of eucalyptus or peppermint oil to the water may speed the process.

Hand, Foot, And Mouth Disease (Coxsackie Virus)

This illness sounds like something you'd get from cattle, but it's actually a common childhood condition that looks worse than it is. Your child may develop a fever, followed by sores inside his mouth and a rash that doesn't itch—usually on the hands, feet, and sometimes the buttocks. It spreads through sneezing, coughing, and other bodily secretions, even though these are not symptoms of the illness. Hand, foot, and mouth disease will resolve and fade away on its own, but in the meantime, you can help reduce your child's discomfort.

WASH, CLEAN, AND DISINFECT

First, do your best to teach your child about hand washing as a preventive to a wide range of illnesses. Clean and disinfect surfaces that may have come in contact with someone who has this illness, and change your bathroom towels after you have visitors, especially those with small children.

SALT WATER RINSE

Dissolve ½ teaspoon of salt in a glass of warm water. Have your child swish this around in his mouth for fifteen to thirty seconds, and spit it out. This will soothe the pain of mouth sores.

DRINK COOL MILK

Milk products are particularly effective in cooling mouth sores and reducing their sting. Have your child drink milk instead of juice or soda, both of which are acidic and will irritate the lesions in his mouth.

PLENTY OF FLUIDS FOR FEVER

Your child may be feverish during this illness, which means that his body will need more water and other fluids to stay properly hydrated. Again, milk and water are your best choices as well as cooling liquids like herbal teas, if your child will drink them. Stay away from sugary or fruity drinks that will irritate the mouth sores. Ice pops, frozen fruit bars, and slushy drinks may be easier for your child to tolerate.

Headache

Psychology Today says that 90 percent of all school-age children get headaches, and that most of these are caused by stress and anxiety. Anyone might get a headache once in a while, but if your child's pain recurs regularly, there may be a larger problem afoot.

AVOID COMMON TRIGGERS

Chocolate, caffeine, sugar, and cheese can all lead to headaches, so limiting these triggers can help reduce the frequency of your child's pain. This does not mean that your child can never have a piece of chocolate again, but you can watch what happens when she has chocolate or cheese and see if a headache follows within a few hours.

KEEP A JOURNAL

When your child comes home from school with a headache or develops one at home, talk to her about what she ate that day and what went on during and after school. Keep notes in a spiral notebook or in an Excel spreadsheet. You may find a pattern that reveals a sensitivity to a specific food—or you may discover a hidden stressor in your child's life that you didn't know about.

DIM THE LIGHTS

Resting in a dark, quiet room can help relieve the headache. Bright lights and loud noises are the worst thing for any headache, and the amount of time children spend looking at smartphones, televisions, and computer screens can make headaches much worse. Rest and sleep can restore normalcy.

When to See a Doctor For frequent and severe headaches, your doctor can help you determine their cause and ways to eliminate the issue. Your child may be facing significant stress—a bully, a problem at school, or any number of issues. The stressor may even be in your home.

Head Lice

When you discover that your child has head lice, you may feel like a terrible parent who is not keeping the child adequately clean. This is not the case—head lice are common among children from every background, in every school, in every part of the country. The appearance of lice does mean that you'll have to remove the lice and prevent them from multiplying.

COAT THEM WITH OIL

Slow the lice down to make them easier to remove with a lice comb.

1. Coat your child's hair with olive or almond oil. Some sources suggest Vaseline or mayonnaise, but these are particularly messy and hard to remove from the hair, and they are no more effective than the oils.
2. Separate the hair into sections, using a comb. Fasten the hair out of the way with hair clips, so you can work on one section at a time.
3. Use a lice comb (available at your pharmacy) to comb through your child's hair to find the lice. Remove the lice with the comb and discard them.
4. Wash your child's hair using her regular shampoo. Rinse and repeat.
5. Dry your child's hair with a towel. Launder the towel right away.
6. Wash the lice comb and any other tools you used by soaking them in vinegar for thirty minutes.
7. Follow these steps every day for a week. After the first week, continue to comb out your child's hair with the lice comb for another two weeks to be sure that the lice are gone.

ALCOHOL SPRAY FOR PREVENTION

Once the lice are gone, put four ounces of alcohol in a spray bottle and spray it on your child's hair at night for two weeks. Use the lice comb to remove any remaining lice and to check for reappearance.

GET THE NITS

Vinegar and water is a common home remedy to help get rid of lice eggs, or nits, though it will not kill the adult lice. Nits are brownish in color but can appear translucent against the scalp. They stick to the scalp and hair like glue, making them especially difficult to get rid of. Follow these steps to help loosen and remove the nits from the hair:

1. Mix white, apple cider (organic), or red wine vinegar and with equal parts water.
2. Soak the hair with the solution for 30 minutes to 1 hour.

3. Use a lice comb to remove every single nit.
4. Rinse the hair after all the nits have been removed.
5. Check your child's head every day for the next 2 weeks to be sure the lice are gone.

Vinegar is nontoxic but can sting the eyes, so you might want to give your child a washcloth to hold against her face during this treatment. For the same reason, do not use this treatment if there are cuts or scrapes on your child's head.

Pinkeye (Conjunctivitis)

The redness, discomfort and discharge associated with pinkeye can be caused by allergies, an eye infection or virus, or exposure to chemicals. The irritant or infection affects the clear membrane covering the white of the eye as well as the membrane on the inner eyelid. If a virus or infection is the cause, your child's case of pinkeye is very contagious—so you will need to wash your hands frequently while treating your child to be sure you don't contract the condition yourself. Wash any washcloths, towels, or clothing immediately that has come in contact with your child's eyes.

If your child has symptoms of a cold or flu along with pinkeye, it's likely that the virus or bacterial infection has caused the eye infection. See your doctor for a prescription for antibiotic eye drops that will cure the pinkeye in a day or so. The remedies below are for pinkeye caused by allergies or other irritants.

A COOL COMPRESS

Clean any discharge or crusts from the eye using a washcloth, and immediately put that washcloth in your laundry. Using a fresh washcloth, wet the cloth with cool water and place it on the eye to soothe the redness and soreness. If the condition affects both eyes, use a different washcloth for each eye. Wash these cloths immediately after using them.

ARTIFICIAL TEARS

Over-the-counter eye drops can go a long way to relieve irritation and bring eyes back to normal. These are inexpensive and safe for children's eyes.

THE BREAST MILK CURE

There's a rumor buzzing all over the Internet about using breast milk to cure pinkeye. While most people will not have this potential remedy available to them, the ones who have tried it—applying a few drops of breast milk to the affected eye—say that it works for their children, particularly for babies. We can only say that there is no scientific evidence to confirm that breast milk is a cure for pinkeye—but there's no proof it isn't, either. If you do try it, be prepared to follow up with your doctor for antibiotic eye drops if you don't see a difference in your child's condition in twenty-four hours.

Sore Throat

When your child complains of a sore throat, you know that this could mean a cold, the flu, a case of tonsillitis or strep throat, or something as simple as too much yelling at the ball game the day before. Whatever the cause, you want to provide relief as quickly as possible.

GARGLE WITH HERBS

Your child may find gargling a little tricky, but once he masters the technique, he'll think it's fun. Create a tea from raspberry leaves (pour a cup of boiling water over two leaves and steep for ten minutes) or from sage (mix one teaspoon of dried sage leaves in one cup of boiling water, and steep for ten minutes). Strain out the leaves and use the warm liquid as a gargle.

Why It Works Red raspberry leaves contain antioxidants that may help relax blood vessels, lessening or eliminating many forms of pain throughout the body. Though still under study, many women use red raspberry tea to help lessen the pain of childbirth. After that, sore throats are a snap.

GARGLE WITH SALT WATER

Your mother was right: There's nothing like this old standby for soothing a scratchy, painful throat and cutting through the phlegm that collects there. Add ½ teaspoon of salt to ½ cup of warm water, and have your child gargle with the solution every three hours.

HONEY AND LEMON

One cup of hot water with one tablespoon of honey and one tablespoon of lemon juice may be just the thing to calm your child's throat. The honey coats the throat and soothes it, while the acidic lemon changes the environment in the throat and may actually help kill the viruses.

When to See a Doctor If your child's sore throat is severe, accompanied by fever or swollen glands, or lasts three days, bring him to the doctor—it could be strep throat. Uncontrolled strep throat can sometimes lead to heart or kidney damage. Strep throat must be treated by antibiotics.

Stomachache

Abdominal pain can take a number of different forms, from stabbing pain to cramps. Many stomachaches can be caused by a child's continued physical development—"growing pains," as they are commonly called—but your child may also have sensitivity to a food group, such as dairy products (lactose intolerance) or wheat (gluten allergy). For the garden-variety tummy ache, here are some effective remedies.

CHAMOMILE TEA

It's not an old wives' tale—chamomile really does soothe the savage beast in your child's stomach. Use a decaffeinated variety, and make one cup of tea from one teabag. Let it cool a bit before giving it to your child.

Why It Works Chamomile has anti-inflammatory properties and it works as a sedative, two qualities that make it an excellent choice for stomach upset. You'll also find chamomile effective as a sleep aid.

GINGER ALE OR TEA

Ginger contains the aptly named gingerol, which acts as an anti-inflammatory that not only relaxes soreness in the intestinal tract, but it also increases the stomach's digestive juices. Drinking ginger ale does indeed assist in clearing up stomachaches, and ginger tea can be even more effective—simply because it contains more ginger and less sugar.

TRY A PEPPERMINT

If your child doesn't like tea, a peppermint candy may do the trick. Peppermint actually increases the flow of bile, a natural substance the body uses in the digestive process. Mint can calm stomach pain and get the digestion back on track.

PROBIOTIC YOGURT

It's not just a marketing scheme; yogurt contains probiotics that replace the good bacteria your child's digestive system may lose in other ways. This is particularly true if your child has just completed a course of antibiotics, which can kill the good bacteria in the body as well as the ones causing the infection. Try a serving of yogurt every day until the stomach trouble passes.

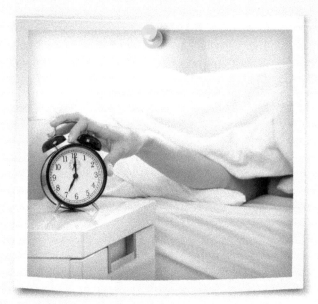

EVERYDAY WELLNESS & GROOMING

- Acne
- Balanced Diet
- Blackheads
- Body Acne
- Body Odor
- Cardiovascular System
- Chapped Skin
- Cracked Heels
- Dandruff
- Dark Under-Eye Circles
- Digestion
- Dry Skin
- Excess Perspiration
- Foot Odor
- Freckles and Age Spots
- Halitosis
- Hair Tangles
- Healthy Hair
- Healthy Skin
- Ingrown Hair
- Liver Function
- Mental Health
- Mood
- Oily Hair
- Puffy Eyes
- Sexual Desire
- Skin Tag
- Sleep
- Spider Veins
- Split Ends
- Splitting Nails
- Stained Teeth
- Stretch Marks
- Teeth
- Thickened Nails
- Thinning Hair
- Wrinkles

CHAPTER 8

Everyday Wellness & Grooming

This book has focused primarily on remedies for when you feel sick, have pain, or need a way to deal with a chronic condition. One of the most important things you can do for yourself, however, is to maintain the highest possible level of health on a daily basis—to help you increase the number of days you feel your best.

Many of the tips in this chapter take you a step beyond common sense. They may even reveal a thing or two you didn't know about the way your own body functions. Everyone may know, for example, that fruits and vegetables are important to good health. But, not everyone understands the new MyPlate guidelines that recommend that three-quarters of every meal come from plant-based foods. You may believe the most effective hair care comes from expensive salon products but have no idea that just as much benefit—if not more—comes from rinsing your hair with apple cider vinegar, a solution that costs pennies on the salon dollar.

When you're having a rough day, you may crave chocolate. It may surprise you to learn that dark chocolate is not only effective in improving your mood but also a healthy addition to a balanced diet. You may also be amused to discover that sugar is not just for treats but also a terrific exfoliating scrub for your skin.

This chapter is loaded with surprises and spot-on advice to help you improve daily wellness and keep your body in top form, just by following a few simple guidelines and tips.

Acne

Acne is characterized by areas of inflamed skin with pimples, scaly redness, and comedones, which are also known as blackheads and whiteheads. It mostly affects facial skin, but in some individuals it affects skin on the neck, back, and chest as well. (For more remedies on how to treat acne that affects other parts of the body, see Body Acne in this chapter.)

MAKE AN ASPIRIN PASTE

To treat a pimple using aspirin, crush one adult aspirin tablet and add a few drops of water to it to make a paste. Apply the paste to the pimple and allow it to dry; then gently wash it off with plain water. This reduces redness and makes large pimples less painful. Repeat the treatment as needed.

APPLY CHAMOMILE TEA

Chamomile tea can ease the irritation of acne. Brew a cup of chamomile tea and remove the teabag. Allow the teabag to cool; then use it to swab your face and other affected areas.

SWAB WITH APPLE CIDER VINEGAR

Apple cider vinegar aids in regulating the skin's pH and can help detoxify, exfoliate, and soften the skin. Mix two ounces of apple cider vinegar with two ounces of water and apply it as a toner to problem areas on your face or body. Store it in a sealed container in the refrigerator for up to two weeks.

SCRUB WITH OLIVE OIL AND SALT

Although you might think oil will worsen acne problems, olive oil actually aids in healing, helping to rejuvenate damaged skin and improve elasticity. Create a quick scrub with a teaspoon of salt and a teaspoon of olive oil. Using circular motions, rub it gently onto your skin, and then wash it away with warm water.

When to See a Doctor When over-the-counter remedies stop working, home remedies don't have desired results, and you're self-conscious about your acne, see a dermatologist. A study in the *British Journal of Dermatology* found acne sufferers can experience the same social and emotional pressures as people with chronic health problems. Don't put yourself through that—get some help for your acne.

Balanced Diet

One of the best ways to stay healthy is to eat a balanced diet. This helps your body ward off common illnesses and chronic disease, and keeps you in a state of equilibrium. Be sure to include a wide variety of natural foods, fruits, vegetables, nuts, and seeds. It's fine to eat the occasional treat, but do your best not to overindulge.

LEARN THE MYPLATE GUIDELINES

The US Department of Agriculture released a new set of guidelines for healthy eating in the twenty-first century. Known as MyPlate, it nearly reverses the guidelines most adults grew up with since the 1950s—which means that many of today's parents and other adults need to relearn what good nutrition means based on today's clearer understanding of the ways our bodies use food. Visit ChooseMyPlate.gov for the details—but in the meantime, remember these basic rules:

1. Make half your plate fruits and vegetables.
2. Make at least half your grains whole grains.
3. Make only a quarter of your plate protein (meats, eggs, cheese).
4. Switch to fat-free or low-fat milk.
5. Choose foods with lower sodium.
6. Avoid oversize portions.
7. Drink water instead of sugary drinks.

HAVE A SMOOTHIE

Smoothies made with fruit and other wholesome ingredients can put you on the fast track to enjoying a better diet that's also convenient. Replace a junk food meal with a filling smoothie once a day to reap healthful benefits and bring your diet back into balance. Either make smoothies at home or pick them up at a shop nearby—just be sure the smoothies don't contain additives or sugar.

SWEETEN WITH STEVIA

One of the best ways to bring balance to your diet is to cut back on sugar. Stevia is a natural sweetener derived from a plant that is a member of the sunflower family. It has no calories and can be bought as a liquid or powder to add to foods and beverages.

Blackheads

Blackheads are openings in the skin that are covered by a mass of skin debris. They can form on any part of your body. Because they are open, they accumulate dirt and debris, taking on the darkened look that gives them their name. While squeezing blackheads can remove them, doing so can push infected matter deeper into the skin and even cause scarring.

SWAB WITH ASPIRIN PASTE

The salicylic acid in aspirin can help break up the dirt and debris that form blackheads. Mash an adult aspirin tablet and mix it with a few drops of water to form a paste. Rub the paste onto blackheads and allow it to remain there until it has dried. Rinse the area with cool water. Repeat this treatment up to three times each week to keep skin clear. Doing so more often may cause dry patches.

LIFT DIRT WITH EGG WHITES

Separate an egg, discarding the yolk or saving it to cook later. Use a fork to whip the egg white and break up its structure. Apply the egg white to your face in a thin layer, making sure not to get any raw egg into your mouth or eyes. Allow the mask to dry on your face for two minutes, and then add a second layer of egg white. Relax for fifteen to twenty minutes while the egg white dries completely and tightens on your face. Gently peel it off; then rinse your face with warm water and pat it dry with a clean towel.

APPLY TOOTHPASTE

To eliminate blackheads and whiteheads, apply toothpaste to the affected area and allow it to remain there for about twenty-five minutes. It may burn slightly as the toothpaste penetrates the clogged pores. Rinse thoroughly. Repeat application daily for up to two weeks or until the blackheads disappear.

Body Acne

Body acne can affect the back, the buttocks, the chest, the stomach, and other areas. It involves clogged pores and may feature a blend of pimples, whiteheads, and blackheads.

HAVE A LIME RINSE

Limes contain flavonoids and vitamin C, both of which disinfect the skin and promote healing. The acid in lime juice helps slough off dead skin cells and dissolve excess oil. Squeeze the juice from three limes into a spray bottle. Stand in the shower while you spritz it onto the affected area and allow it to remain there for ten to fifteen minutes. Then rinse off with cool water. You can use this treatment up to three times each week to help keep body acne at bay.

DAB ON LAVENDER

Lavender essential oil is a powerful natural antiseptic that can help dry up body acne. Simply apply lavender essential oil to the affected areas with a cotton ball and allow it to remain there. Use this remedy each night before bed to help eliminate blemishes.

DAB ON PINK BISMUTH

To shrink a pimple, simply dab some pink bismuth on it with a cotton ball, allow it to dry, wait fifteen minutes, and then rinse the area with cool water. Repeat as needed.

Body Odor

There are several sources of body odor, including bacterial activity on skin and normal excretions, including those produced by the apocrine sweat glands located mostly under the arms.

EAT YOGURT

Eating a cup of yogurt each day can help reduce bad bacteria levels and thus reduce the amount of odor your body produces. Be sure to choose a brand with no added sugar, and make sure the yogurt contains live, active cultures.

DAB ON SAGE TEA

Many people dislike commercially produced deodorants because of the chemicals they contain. If you'd like to try an alternative, consider using sage tea. Put two teaspoons of dried sage in a tea infuser and place it in a teacup filled with boiling water. Cover the teacup with a saucer and allow the tea to steep for at least ten minutes. After it has cooled, use a soft cloth to dab the tea under your arms. Allow it to dry and repeat daily. You can keep your tea in the refrigerator in a sealed container for up to a week.

ELIMINATE BODY HAIR

The purpose of underarm hair and other body hair is to allow body odor to permeate the air around you. Though this bodily function served our human ancestors well, it no longer seems useful. Removing excess body hair will automatically reduce the amount of body odor that rises up into the air around you.

Cardiovascular System

Your heart and lungs are like an engine that keeps your body going. Without a healthy cardiovascular system, all your organs must work harder. This affects your overall health and may even shorten your life span. When looking after your overall well-being, keep cardiovascular health in mind as you make many day-to-day decisions.

GET MOVING, THEN BUILD MOMENTUM

Exercise boosts your heart rate and keeps your cardiovascular system strong and healthy. If you don't exercise now, begin by walking short distances. You might park your car a little farther from your destination and walk the rest of the way, even if it's just across a big parking lot. Over time, increase the amount of physical activity you do, and work your way up to five fun workouts every week. Enlist a friend or family member to exercise with you and find activities you both enjoy. When exercise becomes a habit, you will be glad you made the effort to improve your well-being. By exercising thirty minutes, five times a week, you reduce your risk of heart disease, help keep excess fat from building up on your body, and prevent hypertension, which leads to other complications as you get older.

HAVE A BOWL OF OATMEAL

Have one bowl of oatmeal each morning for breakfast, and you'll be reducing LDL (bad) cholesterol and guarding against high blood pressure—which is good for your heart—plus you will help your body avoid weight gain and type 2 diabetes. Many companies sell products such as snack bars that contain as many oats as a bowl of oatmeal, so if hot cereal isn't your thing or if you tend to be in a hurry in the morning, try one of these instead.

ENJOY A GLASS OF RED WINE

Enjoy a glass of red wine each evening to help prevent heart disease. Research suggests that while the resveratrol in red wine benefits heart health, the alcohol does, too—as long as it is consumed in small quantities. If you like beer or mixed drinks, stick to one beverage per day to reap cardiovascular benefits.

Chapped Skin

Chapped skin often occurs due to exposure to harsh elements. Symptoms include roughness, redness, and even painful cracks. Wear soft, breathable clothing to help your skin heal. If possible, stay indoors and use a humidifier to accelerate the healing process.

CHANGE YOUR BATHING REGIMEN

It's easy to believe that turning up the heat in the shower will make your skin feel better, but that moment of relief is followed by even dryer skin than you had before. Use warm water instead of hot, and choose a mild, moisturizing soap instead of deodorant soap.

MOISTURIZE AFTER BATHING

As you bathe and shower in water, your skin loses its natural moisture. Although this doesn't usually cause a problem, when the air is warm and humid, it can make chapping worse. Use a thick, oil-based moisturizer after bathing or showering, preferably while your skin is still a little damp. Do this daily, and your skin will heal rapidly.

SOOTHE WITH HONEY

Honey helps seal in moisture and heal minor injuries, making it the ideal remedy for severely chapped skin. After showering or bathing, apply a thin layer of honey to any areas of broken skin; then add a thick layer of oil-based lotion or skin cream.

Cracked Heels

Also referred to as heel fissures, cracked heels are a common problem that can become worse during dry, cold weather when skin tends to lose moisture. Usually cracked heels are simply an unsightly cosmetic problem, but in some cases, they can be painful.

SOFTEN SKIN WITH LEMON JUICE

Get two lemons and two shallow bowls, and lay a towel on the floor. Squeeze the juice of one lemon into each bowl. Place the bowls on the towel. Station thick lotion and a pair of socks nearby; then sit in a chair next to the bowls. Place your heels in the bowls, flexing your feet slightly so that you stay comfortable but don't spill the lemon juice. Allow your heels to soak for ten minutes; then remove your feet from the bowls. Slather your heels with lotion and put on the socks. Repeat this treatment every few days, carefully removing dead skin with a pumice stone as it gradually sloughs off.

Why It Works Citric acid provides a natural exfoliator, making lemons a useful agent against oily and dry skin. Be careful not to leave the juice on your skin for longer than overnight as it can cause a reaction—especially if you spend time in the sun.

LOOSEN DEAD SKIN WITH HYDROGEN PEROXIDE

Fill a footbath or basin with a solution made with twelve ounces of hydrogen peroxide and twelve ounces of warm water. Soak your feet in the solution for fifteen minutes. When your feet have dried, use a pumice stone to gently remove the dead skin that has been loosened by the hydrogen peroxide. Afterward, use your favorite foot moisturizing lotion and wear a pair of thick socks to keep the lotion on your heels and to prevent slipping.

A TIP FROM THE COWS

One of the most effective remedies for dry, cracked heels comes from the barnyard—and if you've experienced the pain of heel fissures, you won't hesitate to try this. Bag Balm, a preparation made by the Dairy Association Company, is used by farmers across the country to treat cows' udders for chapping in winter. Smooth the salve on your heels at night and wear a pair of cotton socks overnight. If Bag Balm's odor turns you off, Udderly Smooth Udder Cream, a shockingly inexpensive product available in most drug stores, has been found effective by some users.

Dandruff

Dandruff looks terrible, but it's really just flakes of dead, dry skin from the scalp. Dandruff—also known as seborrheic dermatitis—is often caused by excessive dryness, followed by excess oil production. In some cases, dandruff is complicated by skin fungus.

SOOTHE ITCHING WITH MOUTHWASH

After washing your hair, rinse your scalp with two ounces of mouthwash. Be careful not to use whitening mouthwash, as it contains hydrogen peroxide, which can lighten your hair. The alcohol in the mouthwash will kill any fungus and help alleviate itching. Leave it on for three minutes before rinsing thoroughly with cool water.

MOISTURIZE WITH OLIVE OIL

To restore moisture and relieve flakiness, wash your hair, and then apply ½ cup of olive oil to your scalp, using a basting brush or your fingers to make sure the oil penetrates thoroughly, all the way to your scalp. Massage it in, and then cover your head with a swimming cap, a shower cap, or plastic wrap. Leave the oil on your head for thirty minutes; then shampoo again, scrubbing thoroughly. Dry your hair and style as usual.

TEA TREE OIL TREATMENT

Add a few drops of tea tree oil to the shampoo in your hand before you wash your hair. Massage the mixture into your scalp as you wash. Rinse and style as usual. Tea tree oil is a remarkable soothing treatment for all kinds of skin conditions, including sunburn, rashes, and cooling your eyebrows and legs after waxing.

Dark Under-Eye Circles

Dark circles often form under the eyes because of stress, strain, and fatigue. While they are usually just temporary, they can cause you to look much older than you really are.

TRY A TEASPOON

Place two standard teaspoons in the freezer for ten to fifteen minutes. Remove the spoons and lie down, resting the backs of the spoons under your eyes. Hold them in place until the cool sensation fades.

LIGHTEN WITH LEMON

Cut two thin slices from a lemon. Lie down and place the lemon slices over your eyes, making sure the fruit is in contact with the darkened skin. Leave the lemons in place for fifteen to twenty minutes as you relax and allow your mind to drift.

ROSE WATER FOR A HOME SPA TREATMENT

If you want to feel as if you've just been to your favorite spa, soak two cotton balls in rose water and place them under your eyes. As the puffiness reduces, your dark circles will recede as well. Using almond oil or applying crushed mint leaves below your eyes will provide that same sense of luxurious relaxation.

Why It Works Rose water has anti-inflammatory properties, which soothe irritated skin. Its antioxidants strengthen skin cells and help skin tissue to regenerate. Some evidence suggests that rose water helps decrease damage to the skin's elastin, the fibers that make skin flexible and allow it to stretch.

Digestion

The digestive system plays a vital role in total well-being, transforming the food we eat into energy that keeps our bodies moving and our minds sharp. You can improve digestion by choosing an activity that you enjoy and spending at least thirty minutes each day moving your body. Whether you walk your dog, dance in the living room, or swim laps, you'll find that regular movement helps improve digestion while also benefiting you in a million other ways.

ENJOY SOME STRAWBERRIES

Fiber helps keep things moving, and strawberries are an outstanding source of delicious, natural fiber. Have one cup of fresh strawberries per day and you'll be treating yourself to 4 g of healthful fiber. Boost your fiber intake by eating some fruit or vegetables with every meal, and make the switch to whole grains. You'll soon enjoy improved digestive health.

PEP IT UP WITH PROBIOTICS

You can easily improve overall digestive health by eating yogurt with live active cultures or by taking a probiotic supplement. As a bonus, studies have shown that probiotics also help reduce bad intestinal flora that are associated with excessive abdominal fat. People who take probiotics regularly often find it easier to lose weight.

DRINK MORE WATER

Make sure you are drinking enough water. Water and other liquids help the body extract nutrients from food, and help keep waste moving through your digestive tract. Drink at least sixty-four ounces of water each day and you'll be well on your way to healthy digestion.

Dry Skin

Dry skin can be caused by sun, wind, saltwater, or dry indoor air. Instead of keeping skin hidden, replenish it. You'll stop itching and discomfort in the process.

TAKE A LUKEWARM BATH

Hot water robs skin of its moisture. Instead of taking a hot bath at bedtime, enjoy a lukewarm soak. Apply a thin layer of olive oil to your skin before toweling off; then pat yourself dry with a soft towel. Apply your favorite body lotion, paying particular attention to your elbows, knees, and other areas that tend to be overly dry.

USE ALOE VERA GEL

If you dislike the feeling of oily moisturizers, use aloe vera gel instead. Apply a thin layer to dry skin twice daily.

COCOA BUTTER FOR DOUBLE THE BENEFIT

Cocoa butter not only smells like your favorite dessert, but it penetrates below the top layer of your skin for deeper moisturizing than most synthetic lotions. This fragrant moisturizer comes from the same cacao plant that brings us chocolate, so it's also packed with antioxidants that neutralize the free radicals in your skin, actually preventing some of the impact of aging.

Excess Perspiration

Perspiration is your body's way of cooling itself: As the sweat evaporates, the body's temperature drops. You may also sweat when you are feeling stressed or nervous. But if you feel that you sweat more than normal, try these remedies.

DRINK TOMATO JUICE

Drink a glass of tomato juice each day for at least a week, and you'll notice that you sweat less. Keep drinking tomato juice every day to continue enjoying this benefit.

USE TEA TREE OIL

Because tea tree oil is an effective astringent, it can help reduce sweating. As it is an antifungal, it can help eliminate odor associated with sweat, particularly in areas that tend to smell bad during hot weather. Using a cotton pad, apply a thin layer of tea tree oil to your armpits as well as to your feet and any other body parts that smell funky.

SAGE TEA REDUCES SWEAT

Drinking a cup of sage tea every day can reduce sweating, though it may take up to three weeks before you see results. The taste of sage may not be to your liking, so make yourself a cup of tea with an additional flavor—for example, make your tea with a sage teabag and a chamomile teabag, or with dried sage leaves and mint leaves.

Foot Odor

Stinky feet are caused by the same bacteria that give limburger cheese its characteristic odor. To stop your feet from smelling foul, keep them clean and dry at all times. If that fails, these fast-acting remedies will do the trick.

SWAB WITH MOUTHWASH

The alcohol in mouthwash kills the bacteria that cause foot odor. After washing and drying your feet, soak a cotton ball in mouthwash and use it to swab your feet, paying close attention to the areas between your toes and around your toenails. Allow your feet to dry thoroughly; then apply a dusting of foot powder and put on clean socks.

MINIMIZE MOISTURE WITH BAKING SODA

If your feet have a tendency to sweat, bacteria will keep coming back to haunt you. Keep your feet dry by dusting them with baking soda after washing and drying them each day. Sprinkle a little extra baking soda into your socks and pour it into your shoes, too. This will help eliminate odor while simultaneously drying up any sweat your feet produce.

THE TEA TREE OIL CURE

Tea tree oil has antifungal properties, so swabbing your feet with it not only reduces the odor but also actually kills the bacteria that are causing the odor. This oil brings its own pleasant scent as part of the bargain.

Freckles and Age Spots

Age spots and freckles are simply areas of increased pigmentation. They usually develop on the skin of fair people. You might be born with freckles, but age spots develop as we get older, and can be prevented by avoiding the sun and using sunscreen.

SOUR CREAM FOR LACTIC ACID

Sour milk, sour cream, or yogurt can provide enough lactic acid to lighten and possibly get rid of your freckles and age spots. Apply the sour cream directly on your freckles, and wait a few minutes for it to dry. Don't wash it off with water—instead, wipe it away with a tissue, and then apply your favorite moisturizer. The spots will fade over time.

FADE WITH LEMON JUICE

If you don't want to spring for an expensive fade cream, try using lemon juice instead. The acid it contains may cause slight discomfort as it works, but most people find that it helps lighten or eliminate freckles and age spots. Squeeze fresh lemon juice into a small bowl and apply it to your face with a cotton ball. Leave it on for fifteen to twenty minutes. After rinsing, apply your favorite moisturizer. Repeat this treatment up to three times a week.

APPLY APPLE CIDER VINEGAR

Apple cider vinegar can be applied topically to lighten freckles and age spots. Dab it on right from the bottle. No need to rinse.

When to See a Doctor When is an age spot not an age spot? If your spot is abnormally shaped, larger than others on your body, and more than one color—you may have a skin cancer. Show your spot to a qualified medical professional right away. Melanoma grows fast and spreads quickly.

Halitosis

Halitosis is simply bad breath. This embarrassing problem is sometimes caused by pungent food, but more often than not, bacterial buildup on the teeth, gums, and tongue is the culprit.

SCRAPE YOUR TONGUE

If you brush and floss regularly and still suffer from halitosis, the problem could be bacterial buildup on the back of your tongue. The tongue's rough surface catches tiny particles of food that can sometimes fester, producing a disgusting odor. Buy a tongue scraper and use it every time you brush your teeth. Though your gag reflex may kick in the first few times, you will eventually find that you can go farther and farther back into your mouth, eliminating odor at its source.

CHEW FENNEL SEEDS

If you have eaten spicy food and your breath isn't exactly fresh, chew a few fennel seeds; then swallow them. This will freshen your breath, and the fennel will aid digestion. Drink a glass of water after you finish, swishing slightly if you need to remove any remaining fennel particles from your teeth.

RINSE WITH BAKING SODA

Mouthwash made with ¼ cup of water and ¼ teaspoon of baking soda can help keep your breath smelling fresh. Use it any time you like. Add a drop of peppermint essential oil to enhance the effect.

Hair Tangles

There are times when the wind or a restless night or an evening of wild dancing can leave your hair a tangled mess. Use these simple remedies to untangle hair without causing breakage.

MASSAGE WITH MINERAL OIL

Rub a tablespoon of mineral oil into the knotted area, then use your fingers to untangle it, strand by strand. The mineral oil will eliminate friction and prevent damage.

WARM OIL TREATMENT

Heat some olive oil in your microwave just until it's warm, and massage it into your hair with particular attention to the tangled part. Gather up your hair into a shower cap, and wear the cap for thirty minutes while the warmed oil does its work. After thirty minutes, remove the shower cap and gently untangle your hair with your fingers. Don't use a brush until all the tangles are out, as a brush can make your hair brittle and you'll have a lot of breakage.

UNDO WITH SUNFLOWER OIL

If your hair has a tendency to tangle while you are showering, use a small amount of sunflower oil to help eliminate the tangles and soften hair. Rub $\frac{1}{2}$ teaspoon of sunflower oil between your palms and then apply it to the ends of your hair. Using a wide-tooth comb, start at the bottom of your hair and gently work your way up, easing your way through tangled portions.

Healthy Hair

Believe it or not, your hair can be a sign of your overall health. When you're not getting what you need, your body diverts energy from nonessentials, such as the hair, to your more vital organs. But when everything is healthy and in balance, your hair is also strong and soft. Here are some remedies for helping hair look its best.

TRY A SHOT OF ESPRESSO

To make hair soft and shiny, brew a shot of espresso and allow it to cool to room temperature. Pour it into a clean spray bottle and apply it to your hair, catching drips with a towel. Allow the espresso to remain on your hair for about fifteen minutes; then rinse, dry, and style your hair as usual.

RINSE WITH APPLE CIDER VINEGAR

You can impart body and shine to hair by adding 1½ teaspoons of apple cider vinegar to one cup of cold water and applying it to your hair after shampooing. There's no need to rinse.

Why It Works Commercial hair products can strip away natural oils, leaving your hair dry and in need of conditioner. Apple cider vinegar balances your hair's natural pH level, leaving it soft and shiny. It also acts as an untangler, so you may not need your usual conditioner.

DEFEAT FRIZZ WITH PROTEIN

Mix two egg yolks with a little bit of warm water (not hot—you don't want soft-boiled eggs), and massage the mixture into your scalp and along the shafts of your hair. Gather your hair on top of your head and wrap it in plastic wrap, or put on a plastic shower cap. Wrap a towel over the plastic, and leave all of this on your head for one hour. Rinse your hair in cool water. The additional protein will banish the frizzies that come with humidity and hot weather.

Healthy Skin

The skin is the body's largest organ. It helps keep your temperature constant, and it reflects your overall well-being. Many of the same habits that nourish the rest of your body also benefit your skin: eating right, getting plenty of exercise, and making sleep a priority are three ways you can keep your skin healthy.

IMPROVE CIRCULATION WITH A SUGAR SCRUB

Good circulation helps skin look and feel its best. Improve your circulation by making a simple sugar scrub to use in the shower. Just add two tablespoons of sugar to one ounce of your favorite liquid body wash. Use your hands or a shower puff to scrub your skin, and then rinse your body thoroughly. Follow up with a blast of cold water to tighten and refresh your skin, if you dare.

REDUCE CELLULITE WITH COFFEE

There is no cure for cellulite, but you can reduce its appearance. To reduce the appearance of cellulite, moisten coffee grounds and rub them into the affected area, using plastic wrap to hold it in place. Leave the grounds and plastic wrap on your skin for ten minutes; then take a shower. This is a messy process, so be sure to do it in the bathroom or in another area that won't be difficult to clean up.

TRY A COFFEE OR SUGAR SCRUB

You can use your choice of plain coffee grounds or sugar to make skin smoother, either on your face or on your body. Use ¼ cup of coffee grounds or sugar with ¼ cup of your favorite liquid soap or facial cleanser. Apply it while showering, using light circular motions to scrub your face or body. Rinse well and apply moisturizer or body lotion after toweling off.

SOFTEN WITH HYDROGEN PEROXIDE

For a skin softening hydrogen-peroxide bath, simply draw a hot bath and add two cups of hydrogen peroxide. If you have dark hair, tuck it up in a towel to prevent it from coming into contact with the peroxide, which can lighten hair. Soak in the tub for up to thirty minutes, towel off, and apply your favorite lotion before getting dressed.

REDUCE SHINE WITH CORNSTARCH

Cornstarch is great for absorbing oil on the face. Apply it with a cosmetic sponge or a brush. Allow the powder to sit on the skin's surface for a minute; then gently dust it away.

TONE WITH APPLE CIDER VINEGAR

When diluted with two parts water, apple cider vinegar makes an excellent facial toner. Mix it up in a jar and apply with a cotton ball.

BRIGHTEN WITH PINK BISMUTH

Brighten a dull complexion by soaking a cotton ball in pink bismuth and swabbing it all over your face. Allow this simple face mask to dry for ten to fifteen minutes before peeling it off. Dull, dead skin will adhere to the pink bismuth, revealing fresh new skin underneath. Rinse your face with lukewarm water, pat it dry, and apply your favorite moisturizer.

RUB ON ROSEMARY ESSENTIAL OIL

To improve skin tone, rub a few drops of rosemary essential oil between your palms and apply it to the oily portions of your face.

Ingrown Hair

An ingrown hair occurs when a hair either curls back or grows into the skin sideways. Shaving rough hair can cause ingrown hairs, as can waxing, tight clothing, and breaking off a hair when attempting to pluck it.

LOOSEN WITH SUGAR

Instead of attempting to remove an ingrown hair forcefully, which can cause infection, use some sugar to scrub the area and exfoliate the skin. Rub the sugar in a circular motion, lubricating it with some water or a bit of soap. Rinse your skin after the sugar dissolves. Repeat daily until the hair emerges on its own.

HEAL WITH ALOE

If ingrown hairs are irritated and itchy, you can soothe them with aloe vera gel. Using a cotton ball or pad, apply a thin layer of aloe to the affected area and allow it to dry. Repeat twice daily for three to five days, until the irritation stops.

SHAVE WITH THE GRAIN

You can avoid ingrown hairs by shaving in the direction that the hair grows, instead of against it. For men, facial hair grows downward on the cheeks and jawbone, up on the neck, and straight out on the chin. For women, leg hair grows downward, as does hair in the bikini region.

Liver Function

The liver detoxifies the body, synthesizes protein, and produces a number of important biochemicals that are necessary for healthy digestion. A healthful lifestyle will help improve liver function, and adding some simple detoxifiers can help even more.

DETOX WITH CRANBERRY JUICE

If you have been drinking more alcohol than recommended, you can ease the burden on your liver by drinking cranberry juice. Choose unsweetened organic cranberry juice, if you can, and drink six 8-ounce glasses of it over the course of a day. To enhance the cleansing effect, repeat the treatment for ten days. Be sure to drink plenty of water in addition to the cranberry juice.

NEUTRALIZE TOXINS WITH LEMON

By neutralizing toxins, you can lighten your liver's load. Fresh lemons help the liver produce important enzymes. Lemons also contain high levels of vitamin C, which the body uses to manufacture glutathione, an important compound that neutralizes toxins. Squeeze a slice of fresh lemon into each glass of water you drink during the day to enjoy the greatest benefits.

A DAILY DOSE OF DARK CHOCOLATE

This will make every chocaholic in the world happy—and it should. An ounce of dark chocolate with 85 percent cocoa or higher provides some of the antioxidant protection your liver needs to guard against cirrhosis. Make sure you choose a chocolate with no high-fructose corn syrup, as this substance brings chemicals into the liver that interfere with its normal functioning.

Mental Health

Good mental health is vital to overall well-being. You can feel sad, irritated, angry, or discouraged sometimes and still enjoy good mental health, as long as those negative emotions are balanced by feelings of cheerfulness, good humor, and inner peace. If you think you may be suffering from a serious imbalance, such as depression or an anxiety disorder, seek treatment. There is no shame in looking after your mental health.

CALM WITH CHAMOMILE

Everyone feels anxiety from time to time, and it's perfectly normal. Calm your nerves with a comforting cup of chamomile tea. It contains compounds that bind to brain receptors that soothe the mind.

CHALLENGE IRRITABILITY WITH CHOCOLATE

Hunger can lead to irritability. Eat one ounce of dark chocolate to curb hunger and improve your mood almost instantly. Chocolate just makes you feel good as well.

Why It Works Dark chocolate contains phenylethylamine, the same chemical your brain makes when you're falling in love. This chemical signals your brain to release endorphins, the compounds that elevate your mood.

COMBAT MENTAL FATIGUE WITH LAVENDER

Brain cells can become fatigued, just as muscle cells can. Deep emotional feelings, a heavy mental workload, and high stress are some of the things that can lead to symptoms of mental fatigue; these include sleepiness, a short temper, and limited attention span. When inhaled, lavender essential oil reduces blood pressure and promotes feelings of pleasant relaxation. Place a few drops of lavender essential oil on a cotton ball. Hold it near your nose and inhale deeply for one minute for instant relief. You can get the same benefits by taking a bath with a few drops of lavender essential oil in it, particularly if you do this at bedtime.

Mood

There are many home remedies that can lift you from a low mood to a higher one. The kind of depression for which home remedies can be helpful involves a low, dejected mood and often includes an aversion to physical activity. Sadness, anxiety, hopelessness, excessive worry, and a loss of interest in enjoyable activities are some of the many signs of depression. So are appetite changes, including overeating or loss of appetite, difficulty concentrating, fatigue, and unexplainable aches and pains. If you suffer from serious depression and have suicidal thoughts, seek medical assistance immediately.

TRY ST. JOHN'S WORT

Some scientific evidence reveals that St. John's wort may be helpful in treating mild depression, thought studies continue—and more recent research points to St. John's wort offering the same level of relief as popular prescription drugs. It's not as effective for major depression, however, and it is associated with sensitivity to the sun, gastrointestinal upset, sleep problems, and other negative side effects. It should never be taken alongside prescription antidepressants, and it can interact negatively with some medications. If you take any prescriptions, be sure adverse reactions with St. John's wort are not indicated.

Why It Works St. John's wort contains chemical compounds that can help stabilize neurotransmitters associated with depression. Choose a brand that has been standardized to 0.3 percent hypericin and follow the manufacturer's recommendations for dosage.

WORK IT OUT

Studies have shown that in many cases, exercise can work just as well as antidepressants. When you exercise, your body releases "feel good" chemicals known as endorphins, which promote overall feelings of well-being and can greatly improve your outlook on life. When you notice depression setting in, increase your physical activity level rather than allowing yourself to remain still. Get plenty of regular exercise to reduce the severity and frequency of your depression.

BREATHE IN SOME ESSENTIAL OILS

To improve your mood, try frankincense, lavender, grapefruit, lemon, or sweet orange essential oil. Diffuse some in your home or office, apply a few drops of diluted essential oil to your temples and the back of your neck, or inhale it in a hot bath. Be sure to check chapter 5 to see which oils need to be diluted and which can be used right out of the bottle.

Oily Hair

Sometimes we just can't get a shampoo when we need one. That's when dry shampoos come in handy.

BRUSH IN SOME CORNSTARCH

Add two or three drops of your favorite essential oil to ½ cup of corn-starch to make a wonderful-smelling dry shampoo you can use any time. Cornstarch is great for absorbing excess oil. When using it as a dry sham-poo, apply it to your scalp only. Allow it to sit for up to three minutes; then brush it out of your hair. If you find you've applied too much, you can use a dry towel to rub away the excess.

TRY ARROWROOT

Using ¼ cup of arrowroot, a powder not unlike cornstarch, can be an effective dry shampoo for people with blond hair. Add up to five drops of your favorite essential oil and mix it up with a spoon. Apply the mixture to your roots or to the oily parts of your hair with an old makeup brush. Brush your hair and style it as usual.

COCOA POWDER FOR BRUNETTES

This is not a joke! Mix two tablespoons of cocoa powder into the corn-starch or arrowroot to give yourself a rich, dark, dry shampoo.

Puffy Eyes

Puffy eyes can be a symptom of stress, exhaustion, allergies, and other issues. Inflammation causes the skin around the eyes to swell, causing a heavy, tired feeling around the eyes while making you look less than fresh.

SHRINK WITH SALT WATER

While eating too much salt can contribute to puffiness around the eyes, applying it externally can help shrink the puffiness away. Mix a teaspoon of salt into one cup of warm water. Dip cotton pads in the solution; then lie down and close your eyes. Cover your eyes with the cotton pads, wait ten minutes, and then rinse your eyes with cold water to remove the salt.

REDUCE SWELLING WITH GREEN TEA

Green tea contains caffeine that helps constrict blood vessels and alleviate swelling. Steep two green teabags in boiling water for three minutes and then remove them and allow them to cool until they're just warm to the touch. Lie down with your eyes closed and place the teabags over your eyes. Leave them there for ten to fifteen minutes. When you get up, rinse your eyes with cool water.

HAVE A BANANA

Peel a fresh banana and cut a one-inch section from it. Mash the one-inch section with a fork, eliminating all lumps. (Eat the leftover banana.) Pat the mashed banana under your eyes and lie down for twenty minutes with your eyes closed. The potassium in the banana will help reduce puffiness and the sugar and the moisture the banana contains will soften and smooth under-eye skin.

Sexual Desire

Balancing out the sexual drive between two partners can be tricky, especially if one is highly motivated toward sex and the other is not. Whether you want to increase your desire or decrease it, there are herbal solutions that may help.

CHASTEBERRY

This aptly named tree—also known as vitex—has been known to help reduce sex drive. Its berries have been used since ancient Athens, when women swallowed chasteberry to reduce their sexual desire so they could sacrifice that desire to their gods. Medieval monks used it to help them maintain their vows of chastity. Today women use it to not only reduce sex drive but also regulate the menstrual cycle.

Why It Works *Vitex* (chasteberry) interacts with the pituitary gland to increase secretions of prolactin, a hormone that causes lactation in women and plays a role in sexual desire and gratification. More prolactin reduces sex drive by counteracting the effect of dopamine, which creates sexual arousal.

YOHIMBE

Once a natural supplement and now also a prescription medication, yohimbe comes from the bark of an African tree. As a medication, it is a monoamine oxidase inhibitor (MAOI) used to treat some forms of depression. It has more widespread use as a treatment for sexual dysfunction, as it can correct the inability to achieve orgasm in men, and encourages sexual desire in women. Talk to your doctor about whether this remedy is right for you.

GINSENG

Safe to use on a short-term basis, ginseng has been shown in studies to improve sexual function in men with erectile dysfunction. A cream form of *Panax ginseng* can be used to curb premature ejaculation.

Skin Tag

Skin tags are harmless, but they are unattractive. Small growths of extra skin can be removed with home remedies, but larger ones may need to be excised by a dermatologist.

TIE IT OFF WITH DENTAL FLOSS

Tie a piece of dental floss around the skin tag's base, making it as tight as possible. This method kills the skin tag by cutting off the blood flow to the area. Repeat the treatment if the floss becomes loose. The offending skin tag should fall off within three to six days.

SHRINK IT WITH TEA TREE OIL

Tea tree oil often shrinks skin tags and sometimes encourages them to fall off. Wash and dry the affected area; then add a few drops of tea tree oil to a cotton ball or cotton pad. Place the saturated cotton over the skin tag and secure it with an adhesive bandage. Repeat this treatment daily for up to two weeks.

THE HANDYMAN'S SECRET WEAPON

Cover your skin tag with a small piece of duct tape. Keep the tape on all day, and check to see if the skin tag falls off when the tape loosens. If not, cover it with a new piece. Keep this treatment up for a few days, and the skin tag should dry up and come off with the tape.

Sleep

Sleep is your body's way of recharging its internal batteries. Whether or not you get enough restful sleep affects your well-being just as much as a proper diet, exercise, and other factors. Adults need between seven and nine hours of sleep each night. Without enough sleep, your ability to learn and retain information may be adversely affected. In addition, you may gain weight, suffer from irritability, and be at risk of hypertension. Your stress levels can increase without sufficient sleep, and your immune system may become compromised. Sleep isn't a luxury, it is a necessity. So make it a priority and enjoy better health.

NOD OFF WITH VALERIAN

Tea containing valerian helps you fall asleep and wake refreshed. Have a cup of herbal tea with valerian about thirty minutes before bed each night for a week, and you will notice a big difference in the way you feel. There are several brands available at supermarkets and health food stores.

LIE ON YOUR LEFT SIDE TO EASE NIGHTTIME INDIGESTION

If digestive discomfort keeps you awake at night, try lying on your left side. This positions the stomach below the cardiac sphincter, which leads to the esophagus. Elevate your head with an extra pillow to enhance the relief this sleeping position provides.

STOP SNORING BY LYING ON YOUR SIDE

Snoring—either your own or a bedmate's—can cause you to lose sleep. Snoring happens when the tongue or tissue in the back of the throat impedes the airway. When lying on your left or right side, you will snore much less, or perhaps not at all. You can put a pillow or a tennis ball behind your back to prevent you from rolling over and snoring during the night.

TAKE A FRAGRANT BATH

If you enjoy taking hot baths, add a drop or two of clary sage essential oil to the bathtub, along with one or two drops of lavender essential oil. Inhale the vapors and relax as you prepare to enjoy a peaceful nights' sleep.

Spider Veins

Spider veins are similar to varicose veins but are much smaller. Often caused by long periods of standing, poor circulation, or heredity, these veins aren't just unsightly, they can also be painful.

INCREASE CIRCULATION

Increasing circulation can prevent spider veins from getting worse, and can strengthen the veins so they hurt less. Do some simple leg exercises and walk for twenty minutes each day, and you'll soon notice an improvement.

USE APPLE CIDER VINEGAR

Apple cider vinegar can help reduce the appearance of spider veins. Before showering each day, soak a soft cloth in apple cider vinegar and apply it to your spider veins. Leave it in place for thirty minutes before showering. This treatment works best when applied twice a day for at least eight weeks.

Split Ends

Hair splits lengthwise when it is damaged, causing frizziness and leading to unmanageability and tangles.

GET A TRIM

The best way to eliminate split ends is to have them trimmed off. You can trim your own hair if you like; just cut the same amount off each strand so it looks even. Be sure to use hair scissors, since those designed for paper will just make matters worse.

MOISTURIZE WITH COCONUT OIL

With your fingers, apply a small amount of coconut oil to the ends of your hair and leave it in place for thirty minutes. Wash your hair and use conditioner. Split ends should be more manageable after this treatment.

DEEP CONDITION WITH OLIVE OIL

Warm ¼ cup of olive oil in the microwave or on the stovetop, making sure it is just a little warmer than your own body temperature. Massage it into your hair, cover your head with a towel, and allow the oil to penetrate for thirty minutes. Wash and condition your hair afterward; then comb it and allow it to dry naturally before styling it.

Splitting Nails

Fingernails and toenails have layers that sometimes separate, causing splitting and peeling to occur. Though sometimes just unsightly, this can also be quite painful.

HEAL WITH VITAMIN E

Cut a vitamin E capsule open with a pair of scissors and apply it to your nails and cuticles. Massage it in gently; then use your favorite hand lotion to moisturize. Repeat this treatment daily until your nails grow out.

MOISTURIZE WITH OLIVE OIL

Olive oil is a natural moisturizer that penetrates dry, cracked nails, helping to prevent further damage. Massage your hands and nails with $\frac{1}{2}$ teaspoon of olive oil twice a day to restore moisture.

WEAR GLOVES FOR HOUSEHOLD CHORES

Washing dishes and doing other household chores exposes nails to harsh chemicals that can contribute to splitting and peeling. Wearing gloves eliminates the potential for exposure and helps promote healthy nails.

Stained Teeth

As you get older, your teeth may become slightly discolored due to exposure to coffee, tea, wine, and other dark liquids. Cigarette smoke can also stain teeth.

BUFF WITH BAKING SODA

Buff out stains with baking soda by applying a dab of toothpaste to your toothbrush, and then dipping it in a small amount of baking soda. This mild abrasive will help whiten teeth and make stains disappear over time.

EAT STRAWBERRIES

Strawberries contain a compound that helps to dissolve stains and keep teeth looking their best. Eat your strawberries plain and be sure to chew them very well so they come into contact with your teeth. Enjoy six fresh strawberries a day and keep up the habit to keep teeth stain-free.

REMOVE STAINS WITH ORANGE PEEL

Yellow stains on teeth can be significantly lightened by rubbing the white underside of an orange peel against the stained area. Repeat this treatment daily to lighten tooth stains naturally.

Why It Works Orange peel contains vitamin C and calcium, which whiten teeth naturally. If you rub the peel over your teeth every night, these compounds will work while you sleep to counteract organisms that make your teeth yellow. Do this for several weeks to achieve a real difference.

Stretch Marks

Stretch marks appear when the skin expands rapidly, either due to growth, pregnancy, or weight gain. Sometimes you can't prevent them, but you may be able to lighten them.

MASSAGE WITH COCONUT OIL

If you are pregnant, massage your abdomen and other areas that are expanding with generous amounts of coconut oil. Do this at least twice a day to keep your skin moist and supple, and it is less likely to develop stretch marks.

STAY HYDRATED

Whether you are pregnant or gaining weight, staying hydrated is the best way to protect your skin from the inside out. Drink at least eight 8-ounce glasses of water each day, and drink more if you live in a hot or arid environment.

HEAL WITH LAVENDER ESSENTIAL OIL

If you notice stretch marks forming, apply a thin layer of lavender essential oil to them daily, continuing until they fade. This process may take a month or longer but will provide results.

APPLY MINERAL OIL

To prevent stretch marks during pregnancy, apply mineral oil to areas that typically expand, including the abdomen, the hips and buttocks, and the breasts. Keeping skin moisturized allows it to stretch easily and minimizes the risk of stretch marks developing.

Teeth

A healthy mouth is one of the primary keys to your body's health. Taking good care of your teeth, gums, and tongue makes it possible for you to maintain a healthy diet, take in the fluids you need for hydration, and maintain a high-quality social life with fresh breath.

BRUSH WITH BAKING SODA

Brushing your teeth with sodium bicarbonate—baking soda—can neutralize the acids in plaque while whitening your teeth naturally without expensive polishes and bleaches. You will find that when used properly, baking soda is neither abrasive nor irritating.

1. Take a pinch of baking soda and put it into a small glass or bowl.
2. Add a little distilled or purified water to the bowl, and mix it into the baking soda. You should create a slightly runny solution to reduce the number of granules.
3. Dip your toothbrush into the bowl to get the solution onto your brush.
4. Starting with your molars, brush your teeth. Move on to the facings and the backs of your teeth.
5. If you like, add a little more water to whatever is left in the bowl and rinse your mouth with it.
6. Rinse out your mouth with pure water, as you normally would after brushing.

DRINK GREEN TEA

Studies have shown that people who drink green tea regularly have healthier gums than those who don't. Green tea extract appears to protect the teeth from erosion, the way that fluoride mouth rinse does. It may even stop starchy foods from increasing tooth decay.

BOOST YOUR VITAMIN D

There's a link between gum disease and low levels of vitamin D, a nutrient we used to get by spending plenty of time out in the sun. Now that we understand the sun's link to skin cancer and other health issues, we must get our vitamin D from the food we eat. Eggs, tuna, salmon, and milk all contain this important vitamin.

Thickened Nails

Thickened nails are often a sign of fungus, particularly if the skin around nails is also hard and thick. Though it takes time and patience to resolve this problem, you can use home remedies to help your nails look better.

SOAK WITH LEMON JUICE

Clear up nails by removing any nail polish and then soaking the nails in lemon juice for five to ten minutes. Repeat this treatment every three days until nails are clear. Avoid dark colors of nail polish in the meantime; choose an opaque, light shade to hide your problem while you treat it.

SCRUB WITH BAKING SODA AND PEROXIDE

Create a fizzy nail treatment by combining two tablespoons of hydrogen peroxide with one tablespoon of baking soda. Remove all nail polish and scrub your nails with this solution. Leave it in place for at least fifteen minutes. Repeat this treatment every three days until nails are clear. Avoid dark colors of nail polish in the meantime; choose an opaque, light shade to hide your problem while you treat it.

Thinning Hair

If your hair is thin because of damage, you can help restore it with simple home remedies. If you are suffering from bald patches or are losing hair rapidly, you could have an underlying medical condition. See your doctor to get a proper diagnosis and protect your health.

THICKEN UP WITH EGG

Eggs contain protein, vitamins A, D, and E, and B vitamins that help strengthen your hair and nourish your scalp. Crack an egg into a bowl and beat it with a fork to blend it. Put the egg into your hair, working it in so it covers your entire head and reaches your scalp. Leave it there for five to ten minutes; then rinse it out with cool water.

GIVE HAIR A LIFT WITH BEER

Beer contains sugar that nourishes your scalp, and protein that gives hair a boost. Shampoo your hair as usual and then pour a room-temperature beer into your hair. Leave the beer on your hair for five to ten minutes before squeezing out the excess and toweling dry. The beer smell will evaporate as your hair dries.

Wrinkles

Wrinkles come with normal aging and will worsen with sun exposure and exposure to dry conditions. Stay hydrated to keep your skin firm and try some home remedies to reduce the appearance of wrinkles.

HIDE WRINKLES WITH ALOE VERA GEL

Skip expensive skin plumpers and hydrate your skin with natural aloe vera gel. After washing your face each morning, apply a thin layer of aloe gel and allow it to dry. The malic acid the aloe contains will help to reduce the appearance of wrinkles while keeping skin moisturized.

EXFOLIATE WITH POWDERED MILK

Powdered milk contains alpha hydroxy acid. This compound removes dead skin cells and stimulates collagen production, reducing the appearance of wrinkles and allowing new skin to shine through. Mix ¼ cup of powdered milk with enough water to make a thick paste; then spread it on your face, rubbing it in lightly with circular motions. Allow the paste to sit on your face for ten minutes; then rinse it off with cool water.

RAMP UP THE OMEGA-3S

The same fatty acids that protect your heart can also help you maintain your youthful complexion. Eat more tuna, salmon, halibut, herring and sardines, or almonds, walnuts, sunflower seeds and sunflower oil to increase your intake of omega-3s and help keep your skin healthy. Fish and nuts also contain selenium, a mineral that keeps free radicals from damaging your skin.

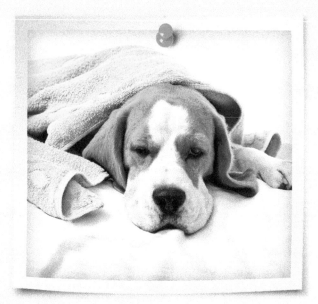

COMMON PET AILMENTS

- Arthritis
- Bad Breath
- Bleeding Nail
- Carsickness

- Chewing Gum in Fur
- Hairballs
- Hot Spots

- Indigestion
- Matted Fur
- Ticks

CHAPTER 9

Common Pet Ailments

We feel so helpless when a loved one is in pain, and that rings doubly true when the loved one is a pet. Animals can't tell you what hurts. In most cases, you will need to visit your veterinarian to be sure that your pet receives the care he needs to feel better . . . but in the short term, it's good to have some options available to bring relief as quickly as you can.

Pets age and grow infirm just as we do, and some conditions become chronic. We can observe joint stiffness, but we can only guess at the pet's pain. We can see discomfort, but it's hard to tell to what extent your dog or cat may be suffering. Having a home remedy for joint pain, upset digestive system, ticks and fleas, and other issues can help you deal with issues that arise again and again, easing your pet's transition from youth to adulthood to his later years just as you would a human loved one.

Arthritis

Like people, pets can suffer from arthritis as they get older. Prescription medications can be hard on internal organs and difficult to get pets to take. Try these home remedies to keep older dogs and cats comfortable.

HEAT THERAPY

Warmth relieves pain and stiffness, helping your pet feel good despite his or her advancing age. Put a soft blanket or a big bath towel into the dryer and get it hot. Give it to your pet to lie on.

A LOW-CALORIE DIET

Pets love to eat, and many of them will eat everything you put in front of them. Choose a diet that offers as much quantity as your pet expects, but with fewer calories and more healthful bulk. Most pet-food makers offer lines of food made for older pets. Try these to reduce your pet's weight to take some of the strain off sore joints.

EXERCISE

Exercise helps pets stay healthy. Encourage your arthritic pet to walk and play in the evenings, after the body has had a chance to warm up. Pets may be more uncomfortable when weather is cold and damp. If they don't feel like moving, allow them to rest and treat them to heat therapy.

When to See a Doctor If nothing you try seems to make your pet any more comfortable, it may be time to try a prescription medication. See your veterinarian to determine the best course of action to give your pet some relief from pain.

Bad Breath

Pets seem to be famous for halitosis. If you notice that Fido or Fluffy's breath is smelling funky, try one or two home remedies to clear the air. But do take your cat or dog for a veterinary check-up, too, because bad breath can be a sign of dental problems.

CARROTS FOR CLEANER TEETH

Boiled or steamed carrots added to your pet's food can help remove plaque from your pet's teeth, defeating one of the causes of halitosis. They also encourage salivation, which will help loosen food particles stuck between your pet's teeth.

PARSLEY TEA KILLS BAD BREATH

Boil some fresh parsley in hot water to make a tea, then wait for it to cool and pour it on your pet's food. Parsley is particularly good for the digestion; a digestive tract issue could be causing your pet's bad breath.

ADD CORIANDER TO TOOTHPASTE

Coriander, part of the cilantro (Chinese parsley) plant, can be added to your pet's toothpaste to kill lingering bacteria in your pet's mouth. Mix in a little from your spice rack before you brush your pet's teeth.

Bleeding Nail

If you regularly trim your dog, cat, bird, or small critter's nails, you know that animals have a quick running through the inside of the nail. The quick is a bundle of blood vessels and nerves. If the nail is white or clear, you can easily see the quick. But if the nail is dark, you can't see it. If you cut the quick, you'll hurt your pet and the nail will bleed a little bit. Avoid causing unnecessary pain by trimming only the very tip of the nail. But if you accidentally do cut the quick, try these home remedies.

SOAP, WATER, AND GENTLE PRESSURE

Wash the cut with soap and water to prevent infection, then wrap the nail, or the entire paw if that's easier, with a clean wet cloth. Gently apply pressure through the cloth to the affected nail until the bleeding stops. If your pet won't tolerate this technique, after washing the nail, try placing a sliver of bar soap on the wound to block the blood flow.

DAB IT WITH CORNSTARCH

Simply dip your finger into a box of cornstarch and then touch the cornstarch to the bleeding nail. It will quickly absorb the blood and form a clump, stopping the bleeding. If your pet later licks it off, cornstarch is perfectly safe.

STYPTIC PENCIL OR POWDER

You may already have this remedy in your medicine cabinet, especially if you've cut yourself while shaving. Applying a styptic pencil or styptic powder to your pet's bleeding nail will stop the blood flow just as well as it does on your shaving nicks and cuts—though it may sting a bit, too.

Carsickness

Many animals love to ride in cars, but travel sickness sometimes stops the fun.

RECONDITION YOUR PET

Dogs and cats are much like people—if something happened the first time they were in the car, they seem to believe it will happen every time. If your pet associates car rides with not feeling well, he may need to be reconditioned to break this association. Try a different vehicle, or take short trips that don't last long enough to cause motion sickness, so your pet has a good time in the car. Treats or toys that he gets only in the car can help make the ride more fun.

Why It Works Just as Pavlov conditioned his dogs to salivate when they heard a bell that they associated with food, you can condition your pet to enjoy a car ride by associating it with something fun. This process takes time and patience, and should be done in small steps.

SNIFF PEPPERMINT ESSENTIAL OIL

Peppermint essential oil can help quickly calm your pet's nausea. Place a few drops on a cotton pad and place it near your pet's carrier in the car. The aroma doubles as a natural air freshener.

TRY SOME GINGER

Natural ginger helps ease nausea in animals, just as it does for humans. You can use ginger essential oil on a cotton ball near your pet, or dab a little ginger essential oil on his or her front paw so that it is near the nose. You can also give your dog a small amount of candied ginger (about the size of the tip of your thumb) thirty minutes before traveling. Hide it in a piece of cheese or lunchmeat if your pet refuses to eat it.

Chewing Gum in Fur

If you have pets and kids, there will be times when chewing gum ends up in your pet's fur. You can simply snip it out with scissors, taking care to keep your fingers between the gum and your pet's skin. If you're worried about cutting your pet in the process, try one of the following home remedies.

EASE IT OUT WITH ICE

Rub an ice cube over the chewing gum until the gum hardens. Use your fingers to crack and break apart the hardened gum. Gently peel off the pieces of gum, making sure not to pull at your pet's hair. When the gum starts to soften, rub another piece of ice on it. Repeat this freezing, cracking, and peeling until all the gum is removed. Then brush the area to remove any remaining residue.

RUB IT OUT WITH PEANUT BUTTER

Gather up a blob of creamy peanut butter in your fingers, and rub it into the chewing gum as well as into the area surrounding it. Leave the peanut butter there for about three minutes. Slide the gum off the hair carefully, and do your best not to tug and hurt your pet. Repeat this process until all the gum is out.

Why It Works The peanut butter contains oils that will make your dog's hair slippery, and will loosen the gum. The oil comes from the peanuts themselves, which are part monounsaturated fats and part polyunsaturated fats. That's why such a sticky substance can unstick a piece of chewing gum.

SLIDE IT OUT WITH OIL

Vegetable oil can help dissolve the gum while also making the process less sticky by coating the gum.

1. Begin by warming up the gum to make it even easier to remove.
2. If your pet can tolerate the noise, set a blow dryer on a low setting and aim it at the gum. Or, warm up the gum with a warm wet cloth.
3. Once the gum is pliable, pour a little vegetable oil into your hand and work it into the gum.
4. Removing small pieces at a time, carefully comb or gently work the gum off the fur with your fingers, massaging more oil into the gum as needed.
5. When the gum is out, be sure to give your dog a bath to completely remove the oil from his fur.

Hairballs

Cats sometimes end up with hairballs that cause discomfort and vomiting. Preventing hairballs won't just help keep your home clean, it will help keep your cat more comfortable.

GROOM YOUR CAT

Cats get hairballs because they swallow hair while self-grooming. One of the best ways to eliminate this problem, and also bond with your cat, is to brush him or her daily to help eliminate loose hair. Use a soft brush and a gentle touch so your pet enjoys the process. Keep the grooming sessions short.

CANNED PUMPKIN

Canned pumpkin contains fiber that helps cats pass hair in their stools instead of vomiting it up on your floor or seat cushions. Give your cat one tablespoon of canned pumpkin (not pumpkin pie filling) each day along with his or her normal food. If your cat needs some encouragement, disguise the pumpkin with a bit of canned tuna juice.

Hot Spots

Dogs get hot spots after a skin irritation causes them to chew and scratch at the affected spot. The chewing and scratching makes the problem worse, causing bacteria to grow and increasing the poor dog's misery. These home remedies will help with the discomfort, though.

COOL WITH WITCH HAZEL

Witch hazel kills bacteria and provides a pleasant cooling sensation. Apply it to hot spots generously, using a spray bottle or a cotton pad. Use this remedy twice daily for up to a week. If you don't see any improvement, your dog could have an underlying problem that calls for veterinary care.

SOOTHE WITH APPLE CIDER VINEGAR

Dab or spray apple cider vinegar onto hot spots to kill bacteria and soothe the itch. Use this remedy twice daily for up to a week. If you don't see any improvement, your dog could have an underlying problem that calls for veterinary care.

When to See a Doctor A veterinary check is the first step in treating a hot spot, because it could be a sign of an internal problem, but also so the hot spot doesn't become worse. Animals often worry a hot spot until they cause an infection.

Indigestion

Pets get indigestion for a variety of reasons. Since your pet can't tell you how he or she feels, you will need to watch carefully to see whether a remedy is helping. Symptoms such as vomiting and diarrhea, which often look like indigestion, can be indicators that your pet is in serious trouble. If problems are not resolved within about twelve hours, get your pet to the veterinarian. The dehydration caused by vomiting and diarrhea can cause your pet's body to shut down rapidly.

WITHHOLD FOOD

If a pet is vomiting or has diarrhea, try withholding his next meal to give his stomach time to settle. Help him stay hydrated by giving him ice cubes or small amounts of vegetable broth. Only withhold food from kittens for four hours.

RICE IS NICE FOR DOGS

Soft-boiled rice can calm a dog's stomach while encouraging normal digestion. If your dog won't eat plain rice, add a small amount of chicken broth. If you dog still refuses to eat, contact your veterinarian. This remedy is not for cats, who do not digest rice very easily.

PLAIN BOILED CHICKEN IS GREAT FOR CATS

Lightly boil skinless chicken breasts in a little water or chicken broth, allow the meat to cool, and chop it up for your cat. Or try some chicken or turkey baby food that was made without onions.

Matted Fur

Long, fluffy hair gives pets a cuddly look and makes them fun to snuggle with, but mats (tangles of fur that gather into clumps) sometimes develop, leading to discomfort and skin infections if left untreated. If your pet has matted fur, do not try to cut the mats out with scissors because you could cut skin trapped inside the mat and cause a serious laceration. Use these simple remedies instead of reaching for the scissors. If your pet has lots of large mats, the simplest course of action is to take him or her to the groomer to be shaved. And then vow to brush your pet regularly so this doesn't happen again.

LUBRICATE WITH CORNSTARCH

Work a tablespoon of cornstarch into the mat and then use a comb to break it up. The starch helps lubricate the tiny hairs, making it easy for you to remove the mat.

SMOOTH WITH CONDITIONER

Work about a tablespoon of hair conditioner into the mat and then use a comb to break it up. The slippery conditioner makes the hairs much easier to work with and helps keep the skin under the mat cool and comfortable.

Ticks

Ticks can cause your pet's skin to become irritated, and some carry serious diseases, including Rocky Mountain spotted fever and Lyme disease. After removing a tick, watch the affected area to be sure no infection sets in. If you have tick-borne diseases in your area, take your pet to the veterinarian even after you have removed the tick. Seal the tick in a glass jar and take it with you. Never crush a tick with your fingernails, as that can expose you to any pathogens it might be carrying.

USE ALCOHOL

Rubbing alcohol helps ease out embedded ticks. Have a helper hold your pet while you pour a little rubbing alcohol onto the affected area. Grab the tick with a pair of tweezers, as close to your pet's skin as possible without pinching the skin, and taking care not to twist or jerk. Pull with steady pressure as the tick backs out.

USE A TICK REMOVER

If you live in an area where ticks are prevalent, invest in a tick removal tool to save yourself time and trouble. You can use this tool on pets and on yourself, should you happen to pick up a tick while enjoying the great outdoors. You can find a tick removal tool for less than five dollars at pet supply stores and online. Follow the instructions that come with the tool to ensure the tick is removed safely. Be sure to do a tick check every time your pet comes in from outdoors, because tick-borne diseases take about a day to transmit. Quick tick removal will prevent them.

Glossary

Abscess An inflamed, infected pocket of tissue filled with pus

Acute Severe, sharp, or intense pain or discomfort; usually brief

Alkaloid Any naturally occurring base containing organic nitrogen; primarily found in plants and plant products

Allicin A pungent compound formed by garlic plants; has antimicrobial properties

Analgesic A substance that eases pain

Antibacterial A substance that destroys bacteria or inhibits its growth

Antidepressant A substance used to relieve depression or treat mood disorders

Antifungal A substance that inhibits the growth of fungi

Antimicrobial A substance that destroys microorganisms or inhibits their growth

Antioxidant An organic enzyme or substance that counteracts damaging tissue oxidization

Antiseptic A substance that inhibits microorganism growth or activity

Antiviral A substance that inhibits virus growth; also any substance that slows or stops the spread of viruses from one person to another

Arterial plaque Cellular waste, fat, calcium, and cholesterol that accumulates on the inner walls of arteries, often leading to blockages and contributing to heart attacks

Astringent A chemical compound that shrinks or constricts tissues

Bactericide A substance capable of killing bacteria

Beta-glucan Dietary fiber found in plants and some mushrooms

Botulinum A bacterial neurotoxin

Bromelain An anti-inflammatory enzyme found in pineapple

Carcinogens Substances capable of causing cancer

Catechins Antioxidant substances found in plants, particularly in tea plants

Chymopapain An enzyme found in papaya; aids in the digestion of protein

Collagen Structural protein that forms connective tissue

COX-2 inhibitors Substances that inhibit COX-2, which is an enzyme that contributes to inflammation

Disinfectant A substance that kills germs or inhibits their growth

Diuretic: A substance that increases urine production

Dyspepsia Difficult, painful, or disturbed digestion; indigestion

Enzymes Proteins that facilitate metabolic processes

Eritadenine A compound that can block cholesterol absorption; found in shiitake mushrooms

Exfoliant A substance that removes dead skin cells from the epidermis

Expectorant A substance that helps loosen and bring up mucus from the lungs, trachea, and bronchi

Flavonoids Plant compounds with anti-inflammatory and antioxidant properties; sometimes called bioflavonoids

Folic acid A water-soluble vitamin that helps the body transform complex carbohydrates into sugars for immediate use as energy

Fracture A broken bone

Histamine A compound released by the human body as part of its natural defense against allergens

Hypnotic A substance that induces sleep

Inflammation The body's response to injury or tissue destruction; often accompanied by pain, swelling, heat, and loss of normal function

Insoluble fiber An effective treatment for irritable bowel syndrome, constipation, and other digestive disorders, fiber that does not dissolve in water; found primarily in grains, fruits, and vegetables

Laxative A substance that promotes bowel movements

Lignans Chemicals derived from various plants including cranberries, tea, flaxseed, and whole grains

Magnesium An element that aids enzyme activity or replenishes electrolytes

Papain An enzyme that breaks down protein; obtained from papaya

Pectin Water-soluble carbohydrates found primarily in fruits

Phenylethylamine A naturally occurring neurotransmitter produced by the brain and found in chocolate and bitter almonds

Phototoxic A substance that makes the skin more sensitive to sunlight

Phytonutrients Nutrients derived from plants

Resveratrol A natural compound that acts as an antioxidant; may protect against cardiovascular disease and cancer

Sedative A substance with a calming, soothing, or tranquilizing effect

Soluble fiber Fiber that is capable of dissolving; enters the bloodstream and clears plaque from blood vessel walls

Stimulant A substance that temporarily accelerates physiological activity

Tryptophan An amino acid that is essential for forming niacin and serotonin; it is formed by proteins during digestion

Vasodilator A substance that relaxes or widens blood vessels; maintains or lowers blood pressure

How to Build a Home Remedy First Aid Kit

Building a first aid kit filled with home remedies involves a minor investment in time and an equally small financial investment. You can make a list, gather supplies, and store your new first aid kit in a safe place within just a few hours, and you won't spend much money in the process.

Begin by determining which injuries and ailments you and your family members and pets are likely to suffer from. Make a list; it's likely that your list will depend on the places you go and the activities you tend to enjoy.

Next, take a look at the home remedies in this book and decide which ones sound most important for your family, based on your list. Make a list of supplies to buy, and gather supplies you already have on hand. While you're at it, get a clear plastic storage bin with a tight-fitting lid, so you can transport your kit when needed.

Finally, add some extra items, including the following, as appropriate:

- Bottle of sterile saline for washing wounds
- Chemical combination thermal/ice pack
- Cotton balls and cotton pads
- Cotton swabs
- Hand sanitizer
- Honey
- Medical tape
- Peppermint tea
- Scissors
- Sealed package of baby wipes
- Sterile bandages in several sizes
- Thermometer
- Tick removal tool
- Tweezers

Make a list of emergency contact numbers and tape it to the underside of the kit's lid. Also make a list of emergency supplies, including prescription medications, that you will need to take with you if you transport your first aid kit.

Check your supplies periodically to be sure nothing has expired. Replace anything that is close to expiring, so your remedies will work when you need them to.

References

American Academy of Pediatrics. "Fewer Infants, Toddlers Harmed by Cough and Cold Medications Since Withdrawal of Infant Products and Label Changes." November 11, 2013. http://www.aap.org/en-us/about-the-aap/aap-press-room/pages/Fewer-Infants-Toddlers-Harmed-by-Cough-and-Cold-Medications-Since-Withdrawal-of-Infant-Products-and-Label-Changes.aspx.

American Cancer Society. "Tea Tree Oil." Last modified November 28, 2008. http://www.cancer.org/treatment/treatmentsandsideeffects/complementaryandalternativemedicine/herbsvitaminsandminerals/tea-tree-oil.

American Pregnancy Association. "Herbal Tea and Pregnancy." Last modified January 2013. http://americanpregnancy.org/pregnancyhealth/herbaltea.html.

Astrup, Arne V., Richard Bazinet, J. Thomas Brenna, Philip C. Calder, Michael A. Crawford, Alan Dangour, William T. Donahoo, et al. *Fats and Fatty Acids in Human Nutrition: Report of an Expert Consultation.* Rome: FAO (Food and Agriculture Organization of the United Nations), 2010.

Attaluri, A., R. Donahoe, J. Valestin, K. Brown, and S. S. C. Rao. "Randomised Clinical Trial: Dried Plums (Prunes) vs. Psyllium for Constipation." *Ailment Pharmacology and Therapeutics* 33. Published electronically February 15, 2011. http://onlinelibrary.wiley.com/doi/10.1111/j.1365-2036.2011.04594.x/pdf.

BabyCenter. "Sleep Problem: Insomnia during Pregnancy." Accessed May 27, 2014. http://www.babycenter.com/0_sleep-problem-insomnia-during-pregnancy_7521.bc.

Bardot, J. B. "50 Ways to Love Your Liver: Home Remedies to Detox and Keep the Life in Your Liver." Natural News. Feb. 22, 2013. http://www.naturalnews.com/039201_live_health_detox_home_remedies.html.

Birk, T., A. C. Grønlund, B. B. Christensen, S. Knøchel, K. Lohse, and H. Rosenquist. "Effect of Organic Acids and Marination Ingredients on the Survival of *Campylobacter jejuni* on Meat." *Journal of Food Protection* 73, no. 2 (Feb 2010): 258–65. http://www.ncbi.nlm.nih.gov/pubmed/20132670.

Brett, Jennifer. "Aloe Vera: Herbal Remedies." HowStuffWorks. January 29, 2007. http://health.howstuffworks.com/wellness/natural-medicine/herbal-remedies/ aloe-vera-herbal-remedies.htm.

Challem, Jack. "A Spoonful of Vinegar Helps the Blood Sugar Go Down." dLife. Last modified December 3, 2013. http://www.dlife.com/diabetes-food-and-fitness/ diabetes-superfoods/special_nutrients/spoonful_of_vinegar.

Chevallier, Andrew. Encyclopedia of Herbal Medicine: The Definitive Home Reference Guide to 550 Key Herbs with All Their Uses as Remedies for Common Ailments. 2nd rev. ed. NY: Dorling Kindersley Publishing Inc., 2000.

"Colds in Children." *Paediatrics and Child Health* 10, no. 8 (October 2005): 493–5. http://www.ncbi.nlm.nih.gov/pmc/articles/PMC2722603/.

Coles, Terri. "Coconut Oil Benefits: 12 Facts about This Wonderful Ingredient." *Huffington Post*. Last modified March 24, 2014. http://www.huffingtonpost .ca/2013/10/25/coconut-oil-benefits_n_4164278.html.

Committee on Health Care for Underserved Women. "Committee Opinion: Oral Health Care during Pregnancy and through the Lifespan." American College of Obstetrics and Gynecologists. August 2013. http:// www.acog.org/Resources_And_Publications/Committee_Opinions/ Committee_on_Health_Care_for_Underserved_Women/Oral_Health_Care_During_ Pregnancy_and_Through_the_Lifespan.

Dehghani, Farzaneh, Ahmad Merat, Mohammad Reza Panjehshahin, and Farhad Handjani. "Healing Effect of Garlic Extract on Warts and Corns." *International Journal of Dermatology* 44, no. 7 (July 2008): 612–5. doi:10.1111/j.1365-4632.2004.02348.x.

Derby, Richard, Patrick Rohal, Constance Jackson, Anthony Beutler, and Cara Olsen. "Novel Treatment of Onychomycosis Using Over-the-Counter Mentholated Ointment: A Clinical Case Series." *Journal of the American Board of Family Medicine* 24, no. 1 (January–February 2011): 69–74. doi:10.3122/jabfm.2011.01.100124.

Fogel, Alan. "Is Your Child Stressed Out? Why You May Not Know." *Psychology Today*. January 7, 2010. http://www.psychologytoday.com/blog/body-sense/201001/ is-your-child-stressed-out-why-you-may-not-know.

Gladstar, Rosemary. Rosemary Gladstar's Medicinal Herbs: A Beginner's Guide. North Adams, MA: Storey Publishing, 2012.

Graedon, Joe, and Terry Graedon. The People's Pharmacy: Quick and Handy Home Remedies. Washington, DC: National Geographic, 2011.

Harvard School of Public Health. "Antioxidants: Beyond the Hype." The Nutrition Source. Accessed January 16, 2014. http://www.hsph.harvard.edu/nutritionsource/antioxidants/.

Healthline. "Rosemary (*Rosmarinus officinalis* Linn.)." Accessed May 27, 2014. http://www.healthline.com/natstandardcontent/rosemary#1.

Heid, Markham. "What Do Probiotics and Oysters Have in Common?" *Prevention*. October 2012. http://www.prevention.com/health/health-concerns/probiotics-shown-help-treat-common-cold%20.

Heinerman, John. Natural Cures for Your Dog and Cat. Edison, NJ: Carol Wright Gifts, 2006.

Javadi, Ezzatalsadat Haji Seid, Fatemeh Salehi, and Omid Mashrabi. "Comparing the Effectiveness of Vitamin B_6 and Ginger in Treatment of Pregnancy-Induced Nausea and Vomiting." *Obstetrics and Gynecology International* 2013. doi:10.1155/2013/927834.

Johns Hopkins Medicine. "Causes of Restless Legs Syndrome." Accessed May 20, 2014. www.hopkinsmedicine.org/neurology_neurosurgery/specialty_areas/restless-legs-syndrome/what-is-rls/causes.html.

Kajiwara, M., and K. Mutaguchi. "Clinical Efficacy and Tolerability of Gosha-Jinki-Gan, Japanese Traditional Herbal Medicine, in Females with Overactive Bladder." *Hinyokika Kiyo* 54, no. 2 (February 2008): 95–9. http://www.ncbi.nlm.nih.gov/pubmed/18323165.

Kaplan, Matt. "Neanderthals Ate Their Greens." *Nature*. July 18, 2012. doi:10.1038/nature.2012.11030.

Keville, Kathi, and Mindy Green. Aromatherapy: A Complete Guide to the Healing Art. NY: Crossing Press, 2009.

KnowYourTeeth.com."How Does Pregnancy Affect My Oral Health?" Academy of General Dentistry. Last modified January 2012. http://www.knowyourteeth.com/infobites/abc/article/?abc=h&iid=325&aid=1309.

King's College London. "Study Shows Acidic Food and Drink Can Damage Teeth." November, 10, 2011. www.kcl.ac.uk/newsevents/news/newsrecords/2011/10October/Study-shows-acidic-food-and-drink-can-damage-teeth.aspx.

Kraft, Sy. "Flaxseed Is King but Won't Help Menopause Symptoms, Breast Cancer." Medical News Today. June 8, 2011. http://www.medicalnewstoday.com/articles/227777.php.

Mallon, Newton, Klassen, Stewart-Brown, Ryan, and Finlay. "The Quality of Life in Acne: A Comparison with General Medical Conditions Using Generic Questionnaires." British Journal of Dermatology 140, no. 4 (April 1999): 672–76. doi:10.1046/j.1365-2133.1999.02768.x.

Mars, Brigitte, and Chrystle Fiedler. The Country Almanac of Home Remedies: Time-Tested and Almost Forgotten Wisdom for Treating Hundreds of Common Ailments, Aches and Pains Quickly and Naturally. Beverly, MA: Fair Winds Press, 2011.

Massachusetts Dental Society. "Canker Sores: A Pain in the Mouth." Accessed May 26, 2014. http://www.massdental.org/cankersores.aspx?id=984.

Mayo Clinic. "Asthma Attack." February 4, 2014. http://www.mayoclinic.org/diseases-conditions/asthma-attack/basics/definition/con-20034148.

———. "Diseases and Conditions: Childhood Asthma." February 8, 2014. http://www.mayoclinic.org/diseases-conditions/childhood-asthma/in-depth/asthma-in-children/art-20044383.

———. "Eyestrain: Prevention." September 19, 2012. http://www.mayoclinic.org/diseases-conditions/eyestrain/basics/prevention/con-20032649.

———. "Nutrition and Healthy Eating." Last updated May 13, 2014. http://www.mayoclinic.org/healthy-living/nutrition-and-healthy-eating/in-depth/caffeine/art-20049372?pg=1.

———. "Tea Tree Oil (Melaleuca alternifolia)." Last modified November 1, 2013. http://www.mayoclinic.org/drugs-supplements/tea-tree-oil/evidence/hrb-20060086.

Medical News Today. "Surprising New Treatment for Childhood Eczema." April 28, 2009. http://www.medicalnewstoday.com/releases/147900.php.

MedlinePlus. "Glucosamine Sulfate." National Institutes of Health. Last modified December 9, 2011. http://www.nlm.nih.gov/medlineplus/druginfo/natural/807.html.

———. "Roman Chamomile." National Institutes of Health. Last modified February 16, 2012. http://www.nlm.nih.gov/medlineplus/druginfo/natural/752.html.

Michels, Alexander J. "Vitamin E and Skin Health." Linus Pauling Institute. February 2012. http://lpi.oregonstate.edu/infocenter/skin/vitaminE/.

Nathan, P. J., K. Lu, M. Gray, and C. Oliver. "The Neuropharmacology of L-theanine(N-ethyl-L-glutamine): A Possible Neuroprotective and Cognitive Enhancing Agent." *Journal of Herbal Pharmacotherapy* 6, no. 2 (2006): 21–30. http://www.ncbi.nlm.nih.gov/pubmed/17182482.

National Association for Holistic Aromatherapy (NAHA). "Exploring Aromatherapy: Safety Information." Accessed May 27, 2014. http://www.naha.org/explore-aromatherapy/safety.

National Center for Complementary and Alternative Medicine (NCCAM). "Chamomile." National Institutes of Health. Last modified April 2012. http://nccam.nih.gov/health/chamomile/ataglance.htm.

National Eye Institutes. "Antioxidant Vitamins and Zinc Reduce Risk of Vision Loss from Age-Related Macular Degeneration." National Institutes of Health. October 12, 2001. http://www.nei.nih.gov/news/pressreleases/101201.asp.

Natural Health Techniques. "Cell Salts." Accessed May 27, 2014. http://naturalhealthtechniques.com/healingtechniquescell_salts.htm.

Nordqvist, Christian. "Coumarin in Cinnamon Causes Liver Damage in Some People." Medical News Today. May 13, 2013. http://www.medicalnewstoday.com/articles/260430.php.

Owen, James. "Neanderthals Self-Medicated?" *National Geographic.* July 20, 2012. http://news.nationalgeographic.com/news/2012/07/120720-neanderthals-herbs-humans-medicine-science/.

Parker-Pope, Tara. "The Science of Chicken Soup." *Well* (blog). *New York Times.* October 12, 2007. http://well.blogs.nytimes.com/2007/10/12/the-science-of-chicken-soup/?_php=true&_type=blogs&_r=0.

Paul, Ian M., Jessica Beiler, Amyee McMonagle, Michele L. Shaffer, Laura Duda, and Cheston M. Berlin. "Effect of Honey, Dextromethorphan, and No Treatment on Nocturnal Cough and Sleep Quality for Coughing Children and Their Parents." *Archives of Pediatric and Adolescent Medicine* 161, no. 12 (December 2007): 1140–6. doi:10.1001/archpedi.161.12.1140.

Pitcairn, Richard H., and Susan Hubble Pitcairn. Dr. Pitcairn's Complete Guide to Natural Health for Dogs and Cats. 3rd ed. Emmaus, PA: Rodale, 2005.

Ragovin, Helene. "Out of Sight." *Tufts Journal.* October 2008. http://tuftsjournal.tufts.edu/2008/10/features/03/.

Rath, Linda. "How Cherries Help Fight Arthritis." Arthritis Today. May 21, 2014. www.arthritistoday.org/what-you-can-do/eating-well/arthritis-diet/cherries.php.

Reader's Digest. 1,801 Home Remedies: Trustworthy Treatments for Everyday Health Problems. Pleasantville, NY: The Reader's Digest Association Inc., 2004.

Reznick, Charlotte. "7 Soothing Remedies for Kids' Headaches." Psychology Today. June 13, 2011. http://www.psychologytoday.com/blog/the-power-imagination/201106/7-soothing-remedies-kids-headaches.

Romm, Aviva. "Ear Infections Part 2: Antibiotics or Natural Remedies for Kid's Ear Infections: What to Use and When." Aviva Romm blog. April 2, 2013. http://avivaromm.com/ear-infections-part-2-antibiotics-or-natural-remedies-for-kids-ear-infections-what-to-use-when.

Rural Spin (blog). "10 Natural Tips for Healthier Hair." March 30, 2013. http://ruralspin.com/2013/03/30/10-natural-tips-for-healthier-hair/.

Sacks, Frank. "Ask the Expert: Omega-3 Fatty Acids." Harvard School of Public Health: The Nutrition Source. Accessed January 16, 2014. http://www.hsph.harvard.edu/nutritionsource/omega-3/.

Schuhmacher, A., J. Reichling, P. Schnitzler. "Virucidal Effect of Peppermint Oil on the Enveloped Viruses Herpes Simplex Virus Type 1 and Type 2 in Vitro." Phytomedicine 10 (2003): 504–10. http://www.ncbi.nlm.nih.gov/pubmed/13678235.

Smith, Tracey J., Diane Rigassio-Radler, Robert Denmark, Timothy Haley, and Riva Touger-Decker. "Effect of Lactobacillus rhamnosus LGG and Bifidobacterium animalis ssp. lactis BB-12 on Health-Related Quality of Life in College Students Affected by Upper Respiratory Infections." British Journal of Nutrition 109, no. 11 (June 2013): 1999–2007. doi: 10.1017/S0007114512004138.

Tiran, Denise. "Is It Safe to Use Essential Oils while I'm Pregnant?" BabyCentre. Last modified July 2013. http://www.babycentre.co.uk/x536449/is-it-safe-to-use-essential-oils-while-im-pregnant#ixzz32hige8D1.

UAB Medicine. "Colds (Chicken Soup)." Accessed May 20, 2014. http://www.uabmedicine.org/news/dear-docs-cold-chicken-soup.

University of Maryland Medical Center. "Low Back Pain." Last modified January 20, 2012. https://umm.edu/health/medical/altmed/condition/low-back-pain

———. "Sprains and Strains." Last modified May 31, 2013. https://umm.edu/health/medical/altmed/condition/sprains-and-strains.

———. "Turmeric." Last modified May 7, 2013. http://umm.edu/health/medical/altmed/herb/turmeric.

US Department of Agriculture. ChooseMyPlate website. Accessed May 4, 2014. http://www.choosemyplate.gov/.

VetInfo. "Home Remedy to Stop Dog Nail Bleeding." Accessed May 27, 2014. http://www.vetinfo.com/home-remedy-to-stop-dog-nail-bleeding.html#b.

Vinegar Institute. "Recent Research Confirms Bactericidal Activity of Vinegar." Accessed May 17, 2014. http://www.versatilevinegar.org/researchnews.html.

Wang, Guangyi, Weiping Tang, and Robert R. Bidigare. "Terpenoids as Therapeutic Drugs and Pharmaceutical Agents." In *Natural Products: Drug Discovery and Therapeutic Medicine*, 197–227. Edited by Lixin Zhang and Arnold L. Demain. Totowa, NJ: Humana Press, 2005.

Warner, Jennifer. "Beet Juice Lowers Blood Pressure." WebMd. December 14, 2012. http://www.webmd.com/hypertension-high-blood-pressure/news/20121212/beetroot-juice-blood-pressure.

WebMD. "The BRAT Diet." Digestive Disorders Health Center. Last modified July 6, 2012. http://www.webmd.com/digestive-disorders/brat-diet.

———. "Cranberries for UTI Prevention." Last modified March 29, 2013. http://www.webmd.com/urinary-incontinence-oab/womens-guide/cranberries-for-uti-protection?page=2.

———. "Cinnamon and Diabetes." Diabetes Health Center. Last modified July 18, 2012. http://www.webmd.com/diabetes/cinnamon-and-benefits-for-diabetes.

———. "Dimethylamylamine." Accessed May 22, 2014. http://www.webmd.com/vitamins-supplements/ingredientmono-1258-DIMETHYLAMYLAMINE.aspx?activeIngredientId=1258&activeIngredientName=DIMETHYLAMYLAMINE.

———. "When to Call a Doctor about Heartburn or Reflux." Heartburn/GERD Health Center. Last modified July 25, 2012. http://www.webmd.com/heartburn-gerd/when-call-doctor.

What to Expect. "Nausea during Pregnancy (Morning Sickness during Pregnancy)." Last modified September 18, 2013. http://www.whattoexpect.com/pregnancy/symptoms-and-solutions/morning-sickness-during-pregnancy.aspx.

Worwood, Valerie Ann. The Complete Book of Essential Oils and Aromatherapy: Over 600 Natural, Non-Toxic, and Fragrant Recipes to Create Health—Beauty—a Safe Home Environment. Novato, CA: New World Library, 1991.

Yahoo! Health. "Pineapple Bromelain." Accessed May 26, 2014. http://health.yahoo .net/natstandardcontent/bromelain.

Zhang, Yuqing, Tuhina Neogi, Clara Chen, Christine Chaisson, David J. Hunter, and Hyon K. Choi. "Cherry Consumption and Decreased Risk of Recurrent Gout Attacks." *Arthritis and Rheumatism* 64, no. 12 (December 2012): 4004–11. http://onlinelibrary. wiley.com/doi/10.1002/art.34677/abstract.

Zirwas, Matthew J., and Sarah Otto. "Toothpaste Allergy Diagnosis and Management." *Journal of Clinical and Aesthetic Dermatology* 3, no. 5 (May 2010): 42–7. http://www.ncbi.nlm.nih.gov/pmc/articles/PMC2922711/.

Ailments Index

Abdominal pain, 124
Achlorhydria, 46
Acid reflux, 102–103
Acne, 40, 56, 71, 82, 88, 94,
    97, 242–243
    body, 245–246
Age spots, 256
Allergies, 32, 35, 37, 97. *See
    also* Asthma
Anemia, 103–104
Anxiety, 43
Appetite suppressant, 28
Arterial plaque, 32
Arthritis, 32, 35, 92, 104–106,
    279–280
    Rheumatoid, 45
Asthma, 32, 106–107, 220–
    221. *See also* Allergies
Athlete's foot, 37, 58, 59, 91,
    107–109

Backache, 200–201
Back pain, 109–110
Bacterial infections, 7
Bad breath, 27, 63, 280–281
Balanced diet, 243–244
Bee stings, 54, 56, 64, 65, 70,
    71, 80, 84, 155–156
Blackheads, 73, 244–245
Bleeding nail, 281–282
Blemishes, 3
Bloating, 36, 45, 47
Blood sugar, 6, 24, 28, 29, 33,
    36, 42, 55, 56
Body aches, 78
Body acne, 245–246
Body odor, 246–247
Boils, 110–111

Bronchitis, 91, 95
Bruises, 3, 80, 111–112
Bumps, 3
Bunions, 112–113
Burns, 6, 17, 37, 54, 65, 70, 84,
    87, 88, 113–114
Bursitis, 114–115

Calluses, 56, 115–116
Cancer, 32, 33, 35–36, 37, 41,
    44, 48
    bladder, 83
    brain, 29
    breast, 24, 32, 39
    cervical, 39
    colon, 24, 32, 35, 39
    gastric, 39
    lung, 24, 29
    ovarian, 35
    prostate, 24, 29, 32, 39
    skin, 29, 39
Canker sores, 63, 91, 117
Cardiovascular disease, 31,
    35, 247–248
Carsickness, 13, 282–283
Cellulite, 3, 60
Chafing, 117–118
Chapped skin, 248–249
Chewing gum in fur, 283–284
Chicken pox, 222–223
Chicken skin, 118–119
Cholesterol, 24, 28, 32, 34, 41,
    42, 44, 48, 69
Colds, 6, 10, 14, 16, 19, 34,
    35, 37, 41, 45, 65, 78, 79,
    82, 83, 87, 90, 91, 94, 95,
    97, 119–120, 210–212,
    223–224

Cold sores, 95, 120–121
Colic, 212–213
Colitis, 122–123
Congestion, 17, 37, 85, 86, 94
Conjunctivitis, 235–236
Constipation, 7, 25, 47, 50,
    88, 123–125, 201–202,
    213–214, 224–225
Copper, deficiency in, 103
Corns, 115–116
Coughs, 37, 46, 65, 83, 90, 91,
    125–126
Cracked heels, 249–250
Cradle cap, 214–215
Crohn's disease, 122–123
Croup, 226–227
Cuts, 54, 61, 87, 88, 126–127

Dandruff, 50, 250–251
Dehydration, 129
Dental pain, 35, 70
Depression, 43, 158
Diabetes, 56, 116
Diaper rash, 69, 215–216
Diarrhea, 17, 25, 50, 70,
    71, 128–129, 216–217,
    227–228
Digestion, 252–253
Dizziness, 202–203
Dry, cracked feet, 40, 65
Dry eyes, 129–130
Dry mouth, 131–132
Dry skin, 65, 253–254
Dyspepsia, 6

Earaches, 5, 132–133
Ear infections, viii, 228–229

Eczema, 40, 93, 133–134, 217–218
Excess perspiration, 254–255
Eyes, dry, 129–130
Eye strain, 134–135
Fainting, 202–203
Fatigue, 135–136
Feet, dry, cracked, 40, 65
Fever, 6, 8, 15, 17, 64, 65, 90, 137–138, 219–220, 229–230
Fever blisters, 120
Fibromyalgia, 138
Flatulence, 138–139
Flu, 10, 14, 16, 34, 45, 82, 83, 87, 140–141, 230–231
Folic acid, deficiency in, 103
Food cravings, 93
Food poisoning, 50, 129
Foot fungus, 58, 63
Foot odor, 255
Frayed nerves, 6
Freckles, 256
Fungal infections, 34

Gallstones, 36
Gas, 36, 47
Gastroesophageal reflux disease (GERD), 46, 102
Gastrointestinal distress, 25
Gingivitis, 69, 172
Gout, 27, 141–142
Gums, receding, 175–176

Hairballs, 284–285
Hair tangles, 257–258
Halitosis, 63, 64, 257
Hallucinations, 158
Hand, foot, and mouth disease, 231–232
Hangover, 142–143
Hay fever, 144–145
Headaches, 3, 15, 16, 17, 19, 46, 86, 88, 93, 145–146, 232–233. *See also* Migraines
Head lice, 233–234
Healthy hair, 258–259
Healthy skin, 259–261

Heart attack, 32, 48
Heartburn, 8, 20, 38, 70, 103, 146–147, 203–204
Heart disease, 33, 34, 44, 48
Heels, cracked, 249–250
Hemorrhoids, 65, 74, 75, 95, 147–148, 204–205
Herpes simplex virus type 1 and 2, 34
Hiatal hernia, 46
Hiccups, 149–150
High blood pressure, 5, 33, 36, 55, 56, 150–151
Hives, 61, 151–152
Hot spots, 285–286
Hyperactivity, 98
Hypoglycemia, 36

Incontinence, 152–153
Indigestion, 6, 40, 45, 46, 57, 70, 85, 86, 90, 153–154, 286
Inflammatory bowel disease, 33
Influenza. *See* Flu
Influenza B, 34
Ingrown hair, 261–262
Ingrown toenail, 154–155
Insect bites, 3, 54, 56, 57, 61, 64, 65, 70, 71, 73, 79, 80, 84, 88, 97, 155–156
Insomnia, 88, 156–158, 205–206, 269–270
Insulin sensitivity, 44
Intestinal cramps, 85
Iron deficiency anemia, 103
Irritable bowel syndrome, 85, 158–159

Joint injuries, 35

Keratosis pilaris, 118
Kidney stones, 39, 159–160

Laryngitis, 74, 75
Leg cramps, 206–207
Liver function, 262–263
Lyme disease, 189

Macular degeneration, 160–161
Malaria, 4
Matted fur, 287
Memory loss, 158
Menopause symptoms, 96, 161–162
Menstrual cramps, 90, 98, 162–163
Mental health, 263–264
Migraines, 32, 49, 163–164. *See also* Headaches
Mini-strokes, 158
Miscarriage, 28
Mood, 264–265
Mood swings, 207–208
Morning sickness, 38, 165–166, 208–209
Motion sickness, 13, 35, 85, 86, 166–167
Mouth, dry, 131–132
Mouth burns, 167–168
MRSA, 34
Muscle aches, 87, 93
Muscle cramps, 81, 168–169
Muscle injuries, 35
Muscle pain, 15, 92

Nail fungus, 169–170
Nausea, 7, 36, 46, 85, 86, 93, 171, 208–209. *See also* Carsickness; Morning sickness; Motion sickness; Seasickness; Vomiting
Nicotine withdrawal, 26
Nosebleed, 171–172

Oily hair, 265–266
Oral health, 209–210
Osteoporosis, 24, 32, 56

Pain
  abdominal, 124
  back, 109–110
  dental, 35, 70
  gums, 172–173
  muscle, 15, 92
  relief from, 7

Pimples, 56, 70, 74
Pinkeye, ix, 235–236
Pneumonia, 83
Poison ivy, 173–174
Premenstrual symptoms
    (PMS), 31, 81, 88, 174–175
Puffiness, 72, 73, 86
Puffy eyes, 266–267

Rashes, 44, 87
Receding gums, 175–176
Reduced cognitive function-
    ing, 158
Restless legs syndrome, 98,
    177–178
Reye's syndrome, 57
Rheumatism, 35, 79
Rheumatoid arthritis, 45
Ringworm, 34, 91
Rocky Mountain spotted
    fever, 188, 189

Scalp itch, 54
Scrapes, 54, 84, 88, 179–180
Seasickness, 13
Seasonal allergies, 180–181
Sexual desire, 267–268
Sinuses, clogged, 15, 19, 97
Sinus pressure, 181–182
Skin
    chapped, 248–249
    dry, 65

Skin tag, 268–269
Sleep apnea, 136
Sore gums, 63
Sore throat, 15, 19, 37, 46, 72,
    73, 74, 75, 83, 84, 85, 86,
    182–183, 236–237
Spider veins, 270–271
Splinters, 184
Split ends, 271
Splitting nails, 272
Sprains, 17, 80, 87, 184–185
Stained teeth, 272–273
Stomachache, 237–239
Stomach cramps, 90
Stomach ulcers, 50
Strains, 80, 87
Strep throat, 83
Stretch marks, 273–274
Stroke, 32, 33, 34, 48
Sty, 185–186
Sunburns, 50, 53, 54, 55,
    186–187
Swimmer's ear, 187–188

Teeth stains, 53
Thickened nails, 275–276
Thinning hair, 276–277
Tick bites, 188–189
Ticks, 287–288
Tinea pedis, 107
Tongue, cleaning, 27
Toothache, 189–190

Tooth decay, 69
Transient ischemic
    attacks, 158
Type 2 diabetes, 28

Under-eye circles, 251–252
Upset stomach, 20, 70
Urinary tract infections, 29,
    191–192

Vaginal dryness, 192–193
Varicose veins, 74, 75, 193
Vitamin B_6 deficiency, 103
Vitamin B_{12} deficiency, 103
Vomiting, 17. See also Car-
    sickness; Morning sick-
    ness; Motion sickness;
    Seasickness

Warts, ix, 194–195
Water retention, 195–196
Wattle tree bark, 4
Whiteheads, 73
Wounds, 37, 84, 97
Wrinkles, 277

Yeast infections, 34, 37, 50,
    196–197

Acetic acid, 128, 186–187
Acupressure bands, 166–167
Ailments
    baby, 210–239
    child, 220–238
    common everyday,
        101–197
    pet, 278–288
    prenatal, 101, 123, 199,
        200–210
Air fresheners, 222
Alcohol, 102, 121, 142, 143,
    152, 288
Alcohol spray, 234
Allicin, 34, 35
Allspice, 7
Almonds, 42, 43, 102, 145
Aloe vera gel, 8, 54–55,
    151–152, 173, 186, 193,
    194, 253, 262, 277
Amino acids, 26
Anbesol, 70
Antabuse, 30
Antacids, 30, 117
Anthocyanins, 138
Antibiotics, 129, 132
    yogurt and, 50
Antidepressants, 31
Antihistamines, 131, 144
Antioxidants, 24, 29, 30, 31,
    34, 48
Antiseptics, 7
Apple cider vinegar,
    55–56, 119, 128, 153–154,
    159–160, 182, 187, 242,
    259, 261, 271, 285
Apples, 24–25, 36, 102,
    146–147

Aromatherapy, 77
Arrowroot, 266
Artificial tears, 130, 236
Asian herb blend, 153
Aspirin, 4, 7, 56–57, 112–113
Aspirin paste, 116, 156, 189,
    190, 242, 244–245
Astringents, 74
Autoimmune diseases, 33
Ayurveda, 7, 69, 138

Baby ailments, 210–239
Baby oil, 66
Baby shampoo, 215
Baby wipes, 174
Bacteria, 15
Bag Balm, 250
Baking soda, 57–58, 103,
    154, 156, 176, 183, 192,
    215, 255, 257, 272–273,
    274–275, 276
Bananas, 24–26, 36, 195, 267
Basil essential oil, 78–79
Bay leaves, 7
BB-12, 120
Beer, 276–277
Beet juice, 150
Behavioral changes, watching
    for, 219
Benzocaine, 70
Beta-blockers, 131
Beta-carotene, 161
Beta-glucan, 44
Bilberry, 161
Birch, 28
Bismuth subsalicylate, 71
Black tea, 106, 136, 164, 181
Black widow spiders, 183

Bleach, 218
Blood thinners, 30, 35, 36, 48
Blow dryer, 132
Blueberries, 191
Blue chamomile essential
    oil, 79
Body hair, eliminating, 247
Borax, 58–59
Borax soak, 108
Boric acid, 59
Boswellic acid, 83
Botulinum spores, 38
BRAT diet, 25, 217, 227
Brazil nuts, 42, 43
Breast milk, 236
Breath, holding your, 149
Bromelain, 47, 105, 114, 122
Bronchi, 106
Bronchioles, 106
Brown recluse spider, 183
Buffing, 118
B vitamins, 26, 40

Caffeine, 59–60, 102, 104,
    106, 136, 152, 164,
    206, 232
Calamine lotion, 223
Calcium, 26, 28, 33, 169
Calcium carbonate, 117
Calendua, 6
Calendula oil, 118
Candida albicans, 196
Carbohydrates, 25
Carrier oils, 78
Carrots, 281
Cashews, 42, 145
Cassia, 29

Cast-iron cookware, cooking in, 104
Castor oil, 111, 124
Catechins, 31
Celery, 26–28
Celery seed extract, 27
Ceramides, 134
Chamomile, 8, 134, 263
Chamomile essential oil, 79–80
Chamomile tea, 153, 238, 242
Chasteberry, 267–268
Cheese, 232
Cherry juice, 138, 157
Chicken, feeding to cat, 286
Chicken soup, 119–120, 140, 211–212
Children
    ailments in, 220–239
    home remedies for, 19
    honey as not recommended for, 38
    safety of home remedies for, 9
Chocolate, 102, 232
    dark, 30–32, 150, 263–264
    milk, 30, 31
    white, 31
Chymopapain, 45
Cinnamon, 28–29, 127
Citric acid, 249
Citrus essential oils, 87
Clary sage essential oil, 81, 163, 175
Cocoa butter, 254
Cocoa powder, 266
Coconut, 128, 159
Coconut oil, 119, 123, 159, 192, 215, 216, 271, 273
Coffee, 59–60, 106, 123–124, 136, 144, 152, 259
Collagen, 24
Complementary medicine, 8
Compress, 185
Condensed tannins, 29
Coneflower, 6
Cool compress, 235
Copper, 161

Coriander, 281
Cornmeal, 170
Cornstarch, 60–61, 118, 126, 216, 261, 266, 282, 287
Corn syrup, 115
COX-2 inhibitors, 27
CRAM diet, 227
Cranberries, 29–30
Cranberry juice, 160, 191, 196, 262
Credit card, 155–156
Cucumbers, 130
Curcumin, 115
Cyanide, 25
Cysteine, 120

Dairy products, 123
Dandelions, 6, 8, 28
Dark chocolate, 30–32, 150, 263–264
Deep breathing, 107
Dehydration, 217
Dental floss, 154–155, 268
Dentist, seeing your, 210
Detoxifying bath, 180
Diaper rash ointment, 118, 222
Dietary habits, home remedies and, 9
Dogs, rice for, 286
Dopamine, 136
Duct tape, 184

Eastern medicine, 125
Echinacea, 8
Eggs, 136, 276
Egg whites, 245
Egg yolks, 259
Electrolytes, 169
Elevation, 184, 193
Enzymes, 41
Epilepsy, 79
Epsom salt, 62–63, 111, 124, 154–155, 169
Eritadenine, 41
Espresso, 258–259
Essential oil diffuser, 79
Essential oils, 8, 78–98
Estrogen, 33

Eucalyptus, 59, 67, 181
Eucalyptus essential oil, 82, 140
Everyday ailments, 101–197
Exercise, 163, 177, 200, 202, 207, 214, 247, 265, 280
Expired ingredients, 9

Feathers, eliminating, 221
Feet, flexing your, 193, 206
Fennel seeds, 257
Fenugreek, 128
Fiber, 24, 25, 26, 28, 32, 43, 102, 124, 175, 201, 225, 252
Fibronectin, 24
Fish, 161
Flavonoids, 31, 40, 74
Flax oil, 32–33
Flaxseed, 32–33
Fluids, 232
Fluoride, 73
Focus, shifting your, 135
Folic acid, 26, 136
Food(s)
    cold, 220
    giving solid, 216
    healing, 23–51
    switching solid, 213
    withholding, 286
Formula, switching brands, 213
Fragrance oil, 78
Fragrant baths, 270
Frankincense essential oil, 82–83, 138, 265
Free radicals, 30
Frozen fruit juice bars, 231
Frozen peas, 172
Fructose, 37, 142
Fur, eliminating, 221

GABA (gamma-aminobutyric acid), 98, 136
Gamma-aminobutyric acid, 98, 136
Gargling, 236–237
Garlic, ix, 33–34, 144, 178, 194–195

Garlic oil, 187
Geranium essential oil,
84–85
German chamomile essential
oil, 79
Ginger, 7, 35–36, 120, 147,
158–159, 167,
208–209, 283
Ginger ale, 165, 238
Ginger essential oil, 85–86,
171, 283
Gingerol, 35, 85, 143, 163, 238
Gingersnaps, 171
Ginger tea, 36, 106, 120, 125,
137, 142–143, 162–163
Ginseng, 268
Gloves, 272
Glucosamine sulfate,
104–105
Glucose, 37
Glycoproteins, 54
Glycosides, 41
Gosha-jinki-gan, 153
Grapefruit essential oil,
86–87, 265
Green tea, 267, 275
Guar gum, 44
Gums, rubbing the, 220

Hair conditioner, 287
Hardy, Karen, 5
Healing foods, 23–51
Heat, 110
Heat therapy, 280
Helichrysum essential oil,
87–88, 140–141
Hemoglobin, 103
Henry VIII, 141
Herbal tea, 165
Herbs, 236
growing, for home
remedies, 11
Hippocrates, 23
Histamine blocker, 24
Homeopaths, 204
Home remedies
from around the
world, 7–8
basics of, 3–11

for children, 19
cost of, 8
defined, 4–5
dietary habits and, 9
expired ingredients and, 9
frequently asked ques-
tions about, 8–11
getting started with,
13–20
growing herbs for, 11
history of, 5–7
methods of using, 14–15
oddness of, 11
overdosing on, 10
purpose of, 8
reasons for not using, 17
safety of, for children, 9
saving, 10–11
scientific support for, ix
side effects of, 9
timing in using, 15–16
tips and techniques for
using, 19–20
use of, with prescription
medications, 8–9
Home remedy first aid kit,
building, 292
Honey, 37–38, 111, 126–127,
142–143, 158, 180, 181,
182, 223–224, 237, 249
Horizon, watching the, 167
Horseradish, 181
Hot bath, 137
Hot compresses, 110–111
Hot showers, 151
Household products, 52–75
Human papilloma virus
(HPV), ix
Humidifiers, 130, 224, 226
Humidity, 132
Hydration, 15, 226, 227, 230,
253, 274
Hydrogen peroxide, 63–64,
74, 108–109, 116, 172, 179,
184, 190, 250, 260, 276

Ice, 64–65, 115, 137, 148,
167–168, 183, 185, 189,
201, 283

Indoles, 38, 39
Insect repellents, 79
Instant iced tea, 174
Insulin, 127
International Federation of
Professional Aromather-
apists (IFPA), 81, 85
Iron, 28, 136
Iron tonic, 205

Journal, keeping a, 233

Kale, 38–39
Kegel exercises, 153

Lactase, 139
Lactic acid, 256
Lactobacillus bulgaricus, 51
Lactose intolerance, 139
Lavender, 6, 59, 67, 77, 156–
157, 177–178, 246, 264
Lavender essential oil,
179, 265, 274
Lemon, 166
Lemon balm essential oil, 90
Lemon essential oil, 89, 265
Lemon juice, 131, 160, 182,
237, 249, 251, 256, 276
Lemons, 39–41, 149, 262–263
LGG, 120
Lice, coating with oil, 237
Lights, dimming the, 233
Lignans, 32
Lime rinse, 245–246
Linalyl acetate, 163
Low-calorie diet, 280
Low-fat foods, 166
Lukewarm bath, 253
Lutein, 160–161

Macaroons, 122
Magnesium, 33, 145
Magnesium sulfate, 62
Maimonides, 119
Malic acid, 44
Manganese, 28, 33
Massage, 135, 207, 225, 229
Meals, eating small, 203

Medical attention, seeking, 18, 19, 20
Mediterranean bay laurel tree, 7
Melissa essential oil, 90
Menthol, 65–66, 74, 93, 109
Menthol rub, 146, 154, 156
Meyer lemons, 40
Milk, 203, 232
Milkweed, 8
Mineral oil, 66–67, 188, 258, 274
Mint, 109–110
"Miracle" remedies, 20
Moisturizing, 249–250
Mold, vanquishing, 221
Motion, 212
Mountain Dew, 106
Mouthwash, 67–68, 108, 112, 131, 250, 255
Mugwort, 28
Multivitamins with iron, 104
Mushrooms, 41–42
Myplate guidelines, 243
Myrcene, 163
Myrrh essential oil, 91–92, 178

National Center for Biotechnology Information (NCBI), 98
Native American people, 8
Natural Medicines Comprehensive Database, 104
Natural oil, 214
Nebulizer, 79
Neti pot, 144–145
Nicotine, 102
Nitric oxide, 150
Nitrogen, 60
Nits, removing, 234
Nonsteroidal anti-inflammatory drugs (NSAIDs), 27
Nuts, 42–43

Oatmeal, 174, 215, 223, 248
Oats, 43–44, 174
Oil pulling, 69

Olive oil, viii, 68–69, 184, 192, 243, 251, 271–272
Omega-3 fatty acids, 32, 33, 186, 207–208, 277
Onions, 7
Orajel, 70
Oral anesthetic gel, 70
Oral health, 209–210
Orange peel, 273
Overdosing, 10

Papain, 45
Papaya juice, 147
Papayas, 44–45
Parsley tea, 281
Pawpaws, 45
Peanut butter, 145, 283–284
Peanuts, 145
Pears, 36
Peas, applying frozen, 105
Pectin, 24, 102
Pedialyte, 143
Peppermint, 46, 59, 67, 77, 146, 151, 158, 238
Peppermint essential oil, 93–94, 109, 121, 136, 164, 283
Peppermint tea, 139, 171
Peppers, eating spicy, 107
Perfume oil, 78
Pet ailments, 278–288
Pharmaceuticals, 4
Phenylethylamine, 31, 164, 264
Phloridzin, 24
Phlorizin, 24
Phosphorus, 40
Phototoxicity, 87, 89
Phytonutrients, 34
Pineapple, 47–48, 122
    bromelain from, 105, 114
Pineapple effect, 122
Pink bismuth, 70–71, 129, 156, 168, 246, 261
Pollen, 37, 38, 180–181
Polysaccharides, 41, 54
Potassium, 25, 169
Powdered milk, 277

Prenatal ailments, 101, 123, 199, 200–210
Prescription medications, use of home remedies with, 8–9
Proanthocyanidins, 29
Probiotics, 50, 120, 129, 239, 253
Prostaglandins, 85, 158–159
Prune juice, 148
Prunes, 148
Psyllium, 148
Pumpkin, 285

Quackery, 6
Quercetin, 24
Quinine, 4

Red raspberry leaves, 236–237
Red wine, 48–49, 248
Relaxation techniques, 205
Rest, 184
Resveratrol, 48
Reye's syndrome, 57
Riboflavin, 136
Rice, 113, 285
Rosemary essential oil, 94, 175, 261
Rose water, 252
Rubbing alcohol, 71–72

Sage tea, 246–247, 254–255
St. John's wort, 264–265
Salicylates, 6–7
Salicylic acid, 71, 244
Saline drops, 211
Saline solution, 224
Salt, 72–73, 243
Saltines, 165
Salt intake, 195
Salt water, 182, 232, 237, 266–267
Sandalwood essential oil, 95, 157–158
Sea salt, 173, 176, 190
Selenium, 33, 43
Sensitive skin products, 133
Serotonin, 136, 162

Sesquiterpenoids, 35
Shaving, 262
Shoes, 109
  sizes of, 112
Shogaol, 35, 85, 143
Sitting down, 202
Sitz baths, 148
Smoking, 227
Smoothies, 26, 28, 30, 36, 47,
  51, 244
Snacking, 165, 208
Sodium, 169
Sodium bicarbonate, 57, 103
Sodium borate, 58
Sodium lauryl sulfate
  (SLS), 117
Sour cherries, 141–142
Sour cream, 256
Soy milk, 161–162
Spices, 206
Spinach, 39
Sponge baths, 219
Sports drinks, 169
Steam, 182, 211, 226, 231
Sterols, 41
Stevia, 244
Strawberries, 252, 273
Streptococcus
  thermophilus, 51
Stretching, 168, 177
Styptic pencil or
  powder, 282
Sugar, 112, 149, 232, 261
Sugarless gum, 131
Sugar scrub, 259
Sulforaphane, 38, 39
Sunflower oil, 258
Supplements, 207
Suppositories, 225
Surfactants, 73
Swaddling, 212
Sweet orange essential oil,
  95–96, 265

Tannins, 74
Tea
  black, 106, 136, 164, 181
  chamomile, 153, 238, 242
  ginger, 36, 106, 120, 125,
    137, 142–143, 162–163
  green, 267, 275
  herbal, 165
  instant iced, 174
  parsley, 281
  peppermint, 139, 171
  sage, 246–247, 254–255
Teabags, 117, 134–135
Tea oil essential oil, 97
Teaspoons, 251
Tea tree essential oil, 179,
  251, 254, 255, 269
Tea tree oil, 113–114,
  170, 176
Teeth, 274–275
Teething ring, 220
Tetracycline, 58
Theobromine, 31
Theophylline, 106
Thiosulfinate compounds,
  34, 35
Thyme tea, 125
Tick, removing, 188
Tissue salts, 204
Tomato juice, 254
Tongue, scraping your, 257
Toothbrushing, 210
Toothpaste, 73–74, 117, 131,
  156, 245, 281
Traditional Chinese
  medicine, 7
Triclosan, 73, 74
Tryptophan, 26
Turmeric, 109, 114–115
Tyramine, 164

Uric acid, 142
Uric acid crystals, 141
Urushiol, 173

Valerian essential oil, 98, 269
Vanilla, 67
Vaporizers, 224
Vinegar, 5, 116, 127–128,
  132–133, 169, 172
  apple cider, 55–56
  soaking feet in, 107–108
Viruses, 15
Vitamin A, 136
Vitamin B_6, 26, 162, 165–166
Vitamin C, 26, 40, 161, 209
Vitamin D, 275
Vitamin E, 126, 161, 168, 272
Vitamin K, 38
Vitex, 267
Vodka, 133

Walking, 139, 150–151,
  162, 208
Walnuts, 42
Warfarin, 35, 36
Warm oil, 228, 258
Warm water, 212
Water, 124, 160, 165, 202, 203
Weight, shifting your, 202
Wellness, using home reme-
  dies in enhancing, 16
White noise, 213
White vinegar, 186–187,
  194, 197
Wild carrot, 28
Willow bark, 6–7
Willow bark extract, 6–7
Witch hazel, 74–75, 121, 151,
  172, 193, 204, 285

Yellow mustard, 113
Yoga, 201
Yogurt, 50–51, 113, 120, 129,
  139, 197, 239, 246
Yohimbe, 268

Zeazanthin, 160–161
Zinc, 43, 161
Zinc chloride, 73
Zingerone, 35

CPSIA information can be obtained
at www.ICGtesting.com
Printed in the USA
JSHW032342030921
18322JS00001B/1